EXCELLENCE IN AMBULATORY CARE

Dale S. Benson, M.D.
Peyton G. Townes, Jr.

("Pursue the Best")

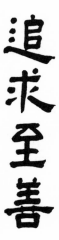

EXCELLENCE IN AMBULATORY CARE

*A
Practical Guide
to Developing
Effective
Quality Assurance
Programs*

Jossey-Bass Publishers

San Francisco • Oxford • 1990

EXCELLENCE IN AMBULATORY CARE
A Practical Guide to Developing Effective Quality Assurance Programs
by Dale S. Benson, M.D., and Peyton G. Townes, Jr.

Copyright © 1990 by: Jossey-Bass Inc., Publishers
350 Sansome Street
San Francisco, California 94104
&
Jossey-Bass Limited
Headington Hill Hall
Oxford OX3 0BW

Library of Congress Cataloging-in-Publication Data

Benson, Dale S.
   Excellence in ambulatory care : a practical guide to developing
effective quality assurance programs / Dale S. Benson, Peyton G.
Townes, Jr.
       p.   cm. — (Jossey-Bass health series)
   Includes bibliographical references.
   ISBN 1-55542-205-5
   1. Ambulatory medical care—Standards.   2. Ambulatory medical
care—Quality control.   I. Townes, Peyton G.   II. Title.
III. Series.
   [DNLM: 1. Ambulatory Care—Standards.   2. Quality Assurance.
Health Care.   WX 205 B474e]
RA399.A3B46   1990
362.1'2'0685—dc20
DNLM/DLC
for Library of Congress   89-26772
                                                              CIP

Manufactured in the United States of America

The paper in this book meets the guidelines for
permanence and durability of the Committee on
Production Guidelines for Book Longevity of the
Council on Library Resources.

JACKET DESIGN BY WILLI BAUM

FIRST EDITION

Code 9013

The
Jossey-Bass
Health
Series

Contents

Preface

A person who sees Quality and feels it as he works is a person who cares. A person who cares about what he sees and does is a person who's bound to have some characteristics of Quality.

> — Robert M. Pirsig,
> *Zen and the Art of*
> *Motorcycle Maintenance*

The discipline known as Quality Assurance is currently receiving much attention in the medical field. Fueled by the rush to cut health care costs, the necessity to ensure adequate quality in care — both to satisfy other professionals and outside accrediting organizations, and to actively provide the best "product" for patients — is creating new challenges for the health care community. Solid Quality Assurance is now being viewed as both the primary means to ensure that quality issues are not pushed into the background by cost considerations and an important way in which providers can protect themselves from malpractice actions.

Quality Assurance can also be a powerful tool in guaranteeing the continuing right of physicians to provide care in ways they select. A long-standing and legitimate tradition of professional medical autonomy has recently begun to clash openly with increasing public demands for individual and organizational accountability. Providers can use Quality Assurance as a mechanism to deliver this accountability while maintaining their right to continue providing care in ways they choose.

Finally, as prepayment programs multiply, the "managed care" cost containment philosophy is becoming more pervasive;

here again, Quality Assurance can be a potent way for health care providers to ensure that quality does not take a back seat to cost reduction.

Purpose of the Book

Even with this growing emphasis on Quality Assurance, there is relatively little information on how to effectively develop such a program in the ambulatory care field—or about how these assessment programs function in the real world. Thus, many ambulatory care managers and providers are unsure of just how to implement valid Quality Assurance. Such uncertainty is a primary reason why we wrote *Excellence in Ambulatory Care*. We intend it to be a genuinely practical tool for anyone involved in the delivery of quality ambulatory health care—from doctors to administrators, nurses to assessment professionals. We believe that everyone working in the development and application of ambulatory care Quality Assurance will find something valuable in these pages.

Because the underlying concepts and broad applications presented here are generic, the book can be used in virtually any outpatient setting: proprietary group practices, hospital outpatient departments, emergi-centers, not-for-profit community health centers, family practice centers, outpatient surgery centers, and so on. It will also be valuable in special types of ambulatory care centers, such as military and government facilities or student health programs.

Excellence in Ambulatory Care is useful from several different perspectives. For those interested primarily in the theory of Quality Assurance, we present a proven model and give detailed descriptions of the various steps necessary to develop a program based on this widely regarded model. For those wishing some insight into directions in which the field of Quality Assurance is likely to move in the future, we have devoted space to both the near term and long-range future of this discipline in the ambulatory care setting. And for those providers and administrators who are in the throes of actual program development or implementation, there are numerous examples from five highly functional Quality Assurance programs in different settings; these study sites can provide practical guidance on how to effectively put quality related theory into daily practice.

Overview of the Book

We have divided this book into three sections, each with its own broadly defined purpose. Part One, "Quality Assurance in Ambulatory Care," describes the role of quality in the ambulatory care field and provides an overview of both the Quality Assurance model we use and the five ambulatory care study sites. In Chapter One, we look at the development of the quality concept in the health care environment (especially in ambulatory care); this view provides some basic perspectives from which a valid Quality Assurance program can be built. Chapter Two presents a generic Quality Assurance model that is a proven approach to implementing a working system. Chapter Three looks at the five sites we visited, each of which gave us excellent program development ideas from its own unique context. (In addition, a description of each site, its structure with respect to Quality Assurance, and some of its important organizational dynamics can be found in Resource A.)

In Part Two, "Key Components in Developing a Successful Quality Assurance Program," we address in more detail the methodology through which Quality Assurance can be made operational. This part essentially parallels the step-by-step process outlined in the proven Quality Assurance model described in Part One. Chapter Four discusses some of the most common objectives of assessment programs in the ambulatory care setting and provides a working definition of quality. Chapter Five deals with the critical issue of gaining credibility for the Quality Assurance effort by appropriately structuring the program within the context of the organization.

We then begin to look at the various components of what is commonly known as "monitoring and evaluation," the ongoing generic process that is central to Quality Assurance implementation. The basic task, as outlined in Chapter Six, is to select what to monitor and evaluate. In Chapter Seven we look at how to develop guideposts against which day-to-day organizational performance can be compared; then we go on to suggest methods for selecting specific criteria and standards. Chapter Eight describes the collection and analysis (through comparison with selected criteria and standards) of performance data in the assessment of organizational quality.

Selection of a unified assessment instrument is the subject of Chapter Nine; we emphasize one specific program that provides a highly structured system for ongoing review and evaluation. Chapter Ten describes how to resolve problems that are uncovered and presents some functional suggestions for ensuring that problems stay resolved. This chapter also offers ways to track the results of Quality Assurance over time so that the overall level of organizational quality continues to improve in practice. In Chapter Eleven, we provide ways to easily formalize program activities through written records, which ensures that Quality Assurance is successfully integrated throughout the entire organization.

Finally, Part Three moves us into the future. Chapter Twelve summarizes the major lessons we have learned both from the proven Quality Assurance model and from our five study sites. The chapter also includes some general principles of Quality Assurance program development and functional "real-world" implementation suggestions. Chapter Thirteen looks at the directions in which Quality Assurance will be moving within the next decade. Chapter Fourteen then takes us to the long-range future of Quality Assurance within the overall health care arena.

In sum, we believe that this combination of solid theory, a proven model, and some practical "how-to" examples will be of significant use to everyone with an interest or investment in the exciting field of Quality Assurance in ambulatory care.

Indianapolis, Indiana   Dale S. Benson, M.D.
December 1989   Peyton G. Townes, Jr.

Acknowledgments

Excellence in Ambulatory Care could not have been produced without major assistance from a number of people. First, we wish to thank the staff at Jossey-Bass, especially Ghila Kapelke, Vivian Koenig, Becky McGovern, Terry Nyquist, Michele Schwartz, and Alis Valencia, without whom we could not have successfully navigated the minefield known as the publishing industry. Their patience in the face of such obstacles as extended deadlines and unending questions (most of which can most charitably be termed "interesting") has earned our sincere respect and gratitude.

Our deep appreciation also goes to the creative and highly committed people at our selected study sites: Frank Houser and Mary Driscoll of Southeastern Health Services in Atlanta; Bruce Biller and Rochelle Alexander of the Massachusetts Institute of Technology Medical Department; Inge Winer of The University of Chicago Hospitals; Magda Cockerline of Washington Outpatient Surgery Center in Fremont, California; and Jane Miller of the Community Health Network, Inc., in Indianapolis, Indiana (our own health center). All of these individuals were kind enough to make themselves and their assessment systems available for scrutiny and open enough to let us shine the spotlight on their programs. All quotations attributed to them were gathered during our interviews for this book.

We also wish to thank the gracious people of Fremont, California; Boston; Atlanta; and Chicago who made our site visits so enjoyable and productive. The hospitality evident in these cities must be experienced firsthand to be fully appreciated. Clearly the Quality Assurance programs within the visitors' bureaus of these cities need little work.

Professionally, we could not in good conscience leave two persons — Avedis Donabedian and R. Heather Palmer — unacknowledged. Quality Assurance in health care owes an immense debt to these groundbreaking theoreticians; their pioneering work is the foundation of both much general Quality Assurance thinking and many of the specific ideas espoused in this book. Donabedian is generally considered the dean of quality assessment in overall health care, while Palmer is one of the earliest and most respected writers on Quality Assurance in the ambulatory care setting. These visionaries deserve our profoundest respect and deepest gratitude.

We also wish to acknowledge the significant contribution of those good friends who provided us with "homes away from home" in various locations and whose generosity made our necessary excursions both uncomplicated and enjoyable. Greg and Iris Clark in Cambridge and Bill and Debbie Stout in Atlanta deserve many thanks for their hospitality. In addition, Skip and Dodie Kappes provided the solitude (in the form of a suitably isolated cabin) that is mandatory for an undertaking of this type, especially in the presence of small children; their contribution also clearly merits our sincere appreciation.

Finally, we owe the deepest gratitude to our wives and families for their steady support, patience, and love. Without their belief in us, our goals, and the necessity of a team effort, this book could not have been written.

Barb Benson has for years kept the home fires burning while her husband flew off in the seemingly never-ending work of refining Quality Assurance ideas. Even at home, her spouse's evenings are often spent at "the little blue desk" as he attempts to make a good thing better. For her patience and understanding, her encouragement and continually positive reinforcement, she is to be commended.

Susie Townes deserves a medal, with love, for her long-suffering patience with that most preoccupied of housemates, a live-in author. Her invaluable contributions included being both mother and surrogate father to an infant and a highly active three-year-old after long days at her own management job and during many distinctly nonrecreational weekends. Suffice it to say that we owe her much.

Finally, we wish to acknowledge the reviewers of our original manuscript. While their identities are unknown to us, many of their suggestions can be seen in the final evolution of this book. Our work is better for their ideas, and we thank them for their contributions.

And so we take up the task of plumbing the sometimes murky depths of Quality Assurance in the ambulatory care setting. But before we get on with the job, we must put the proper perspective on what this book is really about, through two verses from a poem entitled "Why Q.A.?" by Morris Tardiff, the husband of a Quality Assurance professional.

> I fight the battle for Quality Assurance;
> I oft feel my job is a test of endurance.
> Physicians and managers give grudging ear:
> Do they not understand, or just not hear?
>
> Why do I suffer this thankless plight?
> Why do I wage this relentless fight?
> Because of patients I may never see
> Who entrust their quality care to me.

We sincerely hope you find your own involvement with Quality Assurance to be distinctly rewarding—for yourself, for your organization, and, most important, for your patients.

D.S.B.
P.G.T.

The Authors

Dale S. Benson, M.D., is director of Ambulatory Care Services for Methodist Hospital of Indiana, Inc., as well as director of Community Health Network, Inc., a system of three community health centers that serves the inner city of Indianapolis, Indiana. Benson is a Fellow of the American College of Physician Executives and is also certified by the American Board of Family Practice, the American Board of Medical Management, and the National Association of Quality Assurance Professionals.

Benson received his B.A. degree (1963) in chemistry and biology from Greenville College in Greenville, Illinois, and his M.D. degree (1967) from Indiana University. He served his family practice residency at Methodist Hospital in Indianapolis.

Since 1981, Benson has served as field consultant, surveyor, and faculty member for the Joint Commission on Accreditation of Healthcare Organizations. He has surveyed ambulatory care facilities within the United States and as far away as West Germany and Saudi Arabia. Since 1983, he has been a faculty member for Joint Commission seminars both on ambulatory care Quality Assurance and on the Joint Commission's ambulatory care standards. He has also been called upon by the Joint Commission to train new ambulatory care surveyors. He recently served as a member of the task force to revise the Joint Commission's ambulatory care standards.

Benson is on the board of directors of the Society of Ambulatory Care Professionals, as well as a member of the National Health Policy Committee and the National Clinical Directors Sub-Committee of the National Association of Community Health Centers (NACHC). He also serves as a clinical consultant for Region V of the U.S. Department of Health and Human Services (HHS).

His Quality Assurance background is extensive. In addition to his work as faculty for more than fifty ambulatory care Quality Assurance seminars, Benson also serves as a member of several national Quality Assurance task forces, has served as interim director of Quality Assurance for Methodist Hospital of Indiana, and received the 1987 Regional Health Administrator's Award (from HHS) for his development of the AmbuQual Quality Assurance system.

Benson has coauthored numerous professional articles as well as four books on Quality Assurance, including *Quality Assurance in Ambulatory Care* (coauthored with P. G. Townes, Jr., 1987).

Peyton G. Townes, Jr., is currently director of program development for Community Health Network, Inc. (HealthNet) in Indianapolis, Indiana. Prior to that position, he served in a special projects role for the HealthNet system. Townes was also chairperson of HealthNet's Quality Assurance committee for several years during its early development, and during his tenure in this position he developed an active interest in Quality Assurance in ambulatory care.

Townes received his B.A. degree (1969) in English literature from Lehigh University and his M.A. degree (1980) in health care administration from The George Washington University.

He has held several positions in the health care field, including assistant registrar and enrollment representative for The George Washington University Health Plan. Prior to entering the health care field, Townes worked in a professional capacity for the Boy Scouts of America (Norumbega Council) and as an active duty officer in the United States Air Force.

He has worked on several national committees for the National Association of Community Health Centers (NACHC) and served as both secretary and president of the Indiana Primary Health Care Association.

Townes has written or been actively involved with the development of numerous articles, books, and commissioned works both on the health care field and on other topics. His recent published works include *Quality Assurance in Ambulatory Care* (coauthored with D. S. Benson, M.D., 1987).

PART ONE

QUALITY ASSURANCE
IN AMBULATORY CARE

Chapter 1

Improving Quality: The Key to Excellence in Health Care

In the field of health care, we have a long tradition of giving no more than lip service to quality. . . . Clearly, lip service will not suffice. Far more will be sought and even demanded.

—Dennis S. O'Leary,
President, Joint
Commission on
Accreditation of
Healthcare
Organizations

A significant trend is taking place in American business: organizations are placing an ever-greater premium on the quality of their products, and the concept of quality is increasingly being viewed as a "bread-and-butter" issue on its own.

This trend is highly visible in the health care industry, which is particularly appropriate because medicine has a special and undeniable social mission. In the healer's world, what philosophers call the "highest good" has traditionally been no less than the alleviation of human suffering; thus, it is especially important for health care providers to, in the words of an Oriental maxim, "pursue the best."

Unfortunately, while a number of resources document general theories of monitoring, evaluating, and improving quality in the health care field, few attempt to show the daily opera-

3

tion of actual systems that attempt to assure quality. Hence the need for a book such as this.

The Quality Phenomenon

An interesting notion — quality as a phenomenon. Yet one definition of the latter word is "something that impresses the observer as extraordinary" (Stein, 1975, p. 996). In fact, real quality might at first seem to be extraordinary in a corporate environment in which the "bottom line" rules. In such an environment, logic might suggest that actively ensuring goods and services of the highest possible quality would be costly, and therefore counterproductive. However, most successful corporate leaders have never seen things that way. For example, Harold Geneen, who was instrumental in bringing ITT to prominence, believes that "quality is not only right and it is not only free, it is the most profitable product line we have" (Perry, 1981, p. iii).

In truth, it is often much more expensive to fix something than it is to do the job correctly in the first place. A study from the data processing industry pointed out that it was seventy-five times more expensive to make a change after a system's installation than it would have been to make the correct requirement part of the original design (Perry, 1981, p. 10). And, generally speaking, if a feeling of quality permeates a corporate culture, employees will be happier and therefore more productive. In a sense, a spiral builds, with the corporate culture driving the employees, and the employees in turn feeding the corporation and its culture. And everyone comes out a winner.

Another reason why corporate America considers quality to be cost-effective is client satisfaction. The simple truth is that if customers are not satisfied with the quality of a product, they will switch suppliers. And *that* is costly in a very visible way. To validate this, one need only look at the U.S. auto industry in the 1970s and 1980s, when it lost massive sales to foreign manufacturers whose cars had the reputations of being better built.

In predicting the future of American business, John H. Naisbitt, author of *Megatrends*, asserted that "in the new corporation, quality will be paramount" (Gelman, 1985, p. 59). It seems that this prediction was right on target. A company making jeans notes: "Quality Never Goes Out of Style." A dry cleaning chain puts up a billboard announcing: "Quality Spoken Here." Even a spaghetti sauce company puts a "quality button" on its jars to assure the customer that the product is fresh.

In short, quality sells. However, that must be only one concern in any field with a special social mission.

Quality in Health Care

Three related factors form the backdrop for discussions about quality in today's health care field. These are the *cost* of care, the *results* of care, and the client's *perceptions* of care. The idea that quality sells clearly addresses the last issue; cost and results remain. These two issues, and the relationship between them, are at the heart of some of the most dynamic debate currently surrounding health care.

In the 1970s, general alarm started to build regarding the spiraling costs of care in the United States. America now spends more than 11 percent of its gross national product on health care — double the rate being spent just prior to the enactment of Medicare — and costs are still rising. Beginning in the 1970s, broad misgivings began to surface concerning these costs; serious efforts were initiated to slow the upward spiral, and "cost containment," largely through competition among providers (although also through what were termed "voluntary restraints"), became a national watchword. This ardent desire to cut costs has had major consequences, both public and private.

Today, health care providers must actively compete for clients, both individual patients and large groups such as employer insurance plans. The *purchasers* of health care now have much of the economic power and providers are beginning to scramble for the business they once took for granted. And, since these major changes have been driven largely by the cost of care, there is an obvious temptation to compete mainly on price; a second-level temptation is then to cut production costs by providing less service (either in amount or in quality).

Clearly this is not based on the best interest of the patient. Indeed, many providers and theoreticians are highly concerned that the overwhelming focus on cost will lead to serious problems with the results of health care. As a 1988 report to the National Committee for Quality Health Care stated, "Evidence now suggests that cost-cutting policies are cutting beyond inefficiency and threatening availability of services" (Honaker and Robbins, 1988, p. 11).

Partly for this reason, public accountability is increasingly demanded of health care providers; indeed, the very autonomy of the medical profession may be at stake. As a past president of the American Medical Association has noted, the consequence of a lack of vigilance by health care providers could well be a system "in which quality will be lessened, all future medical innovation stifled, and the freedom to exercise professional judgment potentially lost forever" (Boyle, 1985, p. 7).

Such, however, need not be the case. Health care providers of all types are responding in increasing numbers to the mandate for actively preserving quality. The director of the Department of Pathology at Methodist Hospital of Indiana believes, "The eighties will be characterized as the decade when cost became an important factor in health care. The nineties will be characterized as a period when quality will become the predominant issue" (Statland, 1987, p. 3).

A Brief History of Quality Assurance in Health Care

In reality, of course, quality has always been a concern in health care. Although there have been frequent questions about the precise cause-and-effect relationship of specific processes and desired results, practitioners and administrators have shared a need (if not always a desire) to actively review available data and to formulate resulting decisions about the quality of care. Until the early 1970s, the methodology for performing such assessments routinely consisted of individual chart reviews, as well as general evaluation of various discrete statistics (such as mortality data), reports (such as incident reports), or systems (such as personnel systems). There were generally few standard rules or unifying programs; thus, quality assessment largely relied on essentially unstructured reviews of individual events.

Formal Quality Assurance gathered significant steam in the 1970s, partly as the result of the creation by Congress of professional standards review organizations, legal entities that focus on quality review of physician performance by peers. Also during the late 1960s and early 1970s, health care came to be increasingly viewed as more than simply a medical discipline. Growing interest in multidisciplinary models of care resulted in a broadening of ideas about what should be audited for quality; evaluation increasingly involved a variety of health professions, as well as all facets of the patient care process. This signaled a major step forward in identifying the true scope of Quality Assurance.

Simultaneously, the long-recognized health care accrediting organization now known as the Joint Commission on Accreditation of Healthcare Organizations (JCAHO, or the Joint Commission) undertook an initiative to emphasize Quality Assurance in the hospital setting. Part of JCAHO's suggested assessment process involved establishing clear responsibility for Quality Assurance as a key function of the medical staff. (While the same degree of emphasis has yet to be generated in outpatient facilities, formal medical staff organization in ambulatory care organizations is becoming more routine; this will provide an opportunity to increase support for Quality Assurance in this setting, through greater utilization of provider resources in ongoing development of assessment programs.)

Since the early 1970s, Quality Assurance has passed through the following three distinct stages.

First, *medical care evaluation (MCE) studies* involved a specific chart review format that, for accreditation purposes, was mandated on a periodic (for example, quarterly) basis by JCAHO. These MCE studies were, in essence, randomly generated, one-time-only reviews of groups of charts, centering on potential clinical problems. Although they were isolated studies, they did include several improvements over the previous unstructured chart audit system. Perhaps the most important was that each study developed specific criteria that were presumed to have a direct relationship with good patient care. Data were then gathered and compared with preestablished standards based on the selected criteria; any cases that did not meet the standards received more detailed physician review. Unlike the previous medical audits, MCEs allowed reviewers to look for problem patterns in groups of cases.

This stage roughly lasted into the early 1980s; by that time, some problems were being noticed. Since MCE studies were strictly chart based, they were able to assess only the technical aspects of care; therefore, they came to be considered too narrow. They could not, for example, evaluate questions relating to the cost of care or to the interpersonal dynamics underlying the care. And since they depended in large part on physician notes, MCE studies were able to present only one viewpoint. Also, because charts to be reviewed were selected by specific condition, MCE studies could not address the core of the physician's art—skill in making an appropriate diagnosis; indeed, MCE review entirely excluded patients in whom a specific diagnosis had been missed.

And there were other problems as well. Many health care professionals chafed at the requirement to perform a specified number of studies each year using exhaustive criteria that produced massive work loads. Many providers came to feel that such evaluations were often not worth the costs and effort involved. In addition, MCE studies were heavily process oriented, with little real attention to outcome.

Second, the *"problem-finding" phase* lasted from the early to the mid 1980s. This involved a broader but less structured search through as many facets of a health care program as could be comfortably handled, in an attempt to uncover anything that might appear deficient. The operative perspective was, "We think it looks like a possible problem—let's delve into it."

This phase was marked by a less formal approach to assessment; specific techniques for evaluation became less important. It did, however, encourage reviewers to look at a broader range of possible information sources and methodologies. In addition, there was encouragement to integrate all quality-related efforts within an organization into an overall

Quality Assurance program. While this was decidedly useful, an unfortunate consequence was that the program addressed numerous administrative problems, to the extent that these sometimes appeared to overshadow clinical problems.

The real key to problem finding was that the organization had to develop a firm commitment to quality assessment and improvement. However, a lack of concrete guidance on structure and methods, together with the need for greater emphasis on actually solving problems that were uncovered, led Quality Assurance into its next phase in the mid 1980s.

Third, *"monitoring and evaluation,"* as described in Chapter Two, brings us to the present and is now the generally accepted cornerstone of Quality Assurance. It represents a natural evolution from the previous stages, incorporating the structure and periodic nature of MCE studies with the breadth of scope, mandate for commitment to quality, and integration of activities found in the problem-finding stage. This approach pays greater attention to specifying indicators of quality, ensuring that a clinical focus is not overshadowed by administrative issues, and formalizing a rigorous problem resolution process.

This, incidentally, is the model currently being advanced by JCAHO. The Joint Commission has been in the forefront of the field for some time, continually refining the conceptual base on which the discipline is founded. Thus, many consider this organization the expert source on Quality Assurance matters, as well as the primary accrediting body for organizations in the ambulatory health care field. (Several other national organizations also provide accrediting functions and Quality Assurance leadership for ambulatory care organizations; among these are the Accreditation Association for Ambulatory Health Care [AAAHC] and the National Committee on Quality Assurance [NCQA], which serves primarily prepaid organizations.) An increasing number of ambulatory care organizations are now seeking accreditation; for example, all of the organizations we identified as having highly functional Quality Assurance systems (described in Chapter Three and referenced throughout this book) are accredited by JCAHO.

The Ambulatory Care Arena

The field of health care is currently undergoing perhaps the most significant set of changes of the past half-century. A major player in this upheaval is ambulatory care.

With new payment philosophies and alternative providers, there is now a general incentive in the health care industry to keep people out of the hospital. Very simply, ambulatory care is less expensive. At the same time, there is a growing consensus that, if quality is the same, it is also good for the *patients* to receive more of their care in the outpatient setting; if medical conditions can be either prevented through education or screened and treated early, there will be less need to seek inpatient care.

Recent statistics bear out the growing emphasis on — and investment in — ambulatory care. A survey by *Hospitals* magazine found that nearly 80 percent of 2,200 hospitals contacted were actively planning to expand their ambulatory care services (Howard and Newald, 1987, p. 74). Another article (Morrow, 1988, p. 19) quotes John Henderson, a health care researcher, with respect to outpatient surgery centers: "The industry is just taking off." The number of HMOs/managed care plans jumped from 280 in 1983 to more than 660 as of June 1987 (telephone conversation with Nina Lane, Group Health Association of America, October 1988). And the money spent on hospital ambulatory care projects in a recent year caused *Hospitals* magazine to assert, "The trend toward ambulatory care construction is staggering" (Cherskov, 1987, p. 58).

Accompanying this growth in outpatient services is a simultaneous decrease in inpatient hospital days. Both total admissions and overall lengths of stay have decreased during the 1980s; one health care author (Coile, 1986, p. 16) has noted his belief that by the turn of the next century, "the business of hospitals will be redefined 50:50 inpatient-outpatient."

What does all of this portend for ambulatory care? Obviously, the future is bright; ambulatory care is becoming a "boom industry." But along with this comes a concomitant responsibility to take a major role in preserving ethical values in health care—to be in the vanguard of those who "pursue the best."

The task will be far from easy. The assurance of quality in any portion of the health care field is tough; we would argue that it may be even tougher in the ambulatory care setting than in an inpatient environment. The ambulatory care organization must, in fact, deal with a number of complexities that are foreign to the inpatient environment.

First, the outcome in ambulatory care is both ill-defined and relatively more difficult to influence than in the inpatient setting. The ambulatory care provider sees a large percentage of self-limiting diseases, as well as chronic conditions in which treatment is often palliative. In general, the natural histories of many conditions seen in this setting are either poorly understood or difficult to directly affect; thus, measuring the results of care becomes highly complex.

Second, the ambulatory care provider has less control over the patient and the treatment course than does the inpatient provider. Ambulatory care visits are generated by the patient, not the physician (as with a hospital admission); it is also unfortunately true that the patient generally controls compliance with treatment regimens, changes in life-style, and continued exposure to detrimental influences or substances.

Third, the ambulatory patient's total care may be highly fragmented among several providers, and coordination of care is thus a significant issue.

Fourth, the nature of both ambulatory care and ambulatory conditions mandates that rather than confine assessment to a single episode of care, a reviewer must look at conditions and treatments that stretch over long periods of time. Thus, defining the actual "unit" of ambulatory care becomes difficult.

And fifth, there is added importance to what we will call the "art of care" (that is, the quality of the doctor-patient relationship, as opposed to the more technical process, or "science of care," that is often transcendent in the inpatient environment). The provider's ability to get inside the patient's mind to develop a real rapport, thereby motivating the patient, is critical but complex. It is made even more difficult by two factors: the various roles the ambulatory care provider must often fulfill, and the definition of "health" within which such providers must work.

The ambulatory care provider, because of the very nature of the problems encountered, must be a great many things to the patient. Some of the roles the ambulatory care provider is routinely called upon to fill include diagnostician, therapist, guide to other social services, advocate for the patient within those other services, case finder, disease preventer, psychotherapist, health educator, and manager of a total health care team (Palmer, 1983, p. 41).

The way in which the ambulatory care provider must define health is another confounding factor. The schematic diagram shown in Figure 1 may be helpful in conceptualizing the total spectrum of health. At the far left of our "bow tie" diagram is what we will term "total sickness"; the far right side is "total health." It is important to note that, when moving from left to right, "basic wellness" (the simple absence of disease) is encountered at the midpoint, long before "total health" is reached.

The ambulatory care provider's direct responsibility often extends well into the left side of the bow tie, to the secondary care level. As the level of health increases, we move through primary care (often equated with ambulatory care), and into wellness. From here we move into a rapidly developing area of primary/ambulatory medicine, which we will refer to as "positive wellness"; we can further divide this area into "preventive health measures," periodic checkups, immunizations, use of seat belts, and so forth, and "constructive health measures," such as physical fitness programs, nutrition counseling, and stress reduction. The goal in health care at all levels is, of course, to move the patient as far to the right of the spectrum as possible, given the available resources.

Note that the vertical dimension of Figure 1 compresses toward the middle of the bow tie, and expands at both ends. This dimension simply represents the amount of energy, time, money, or other resources required to move farther toward the right in the spectrum of health. Thus, tertiary care consumes an enor-

Figure 1. The Spectrum of Health.

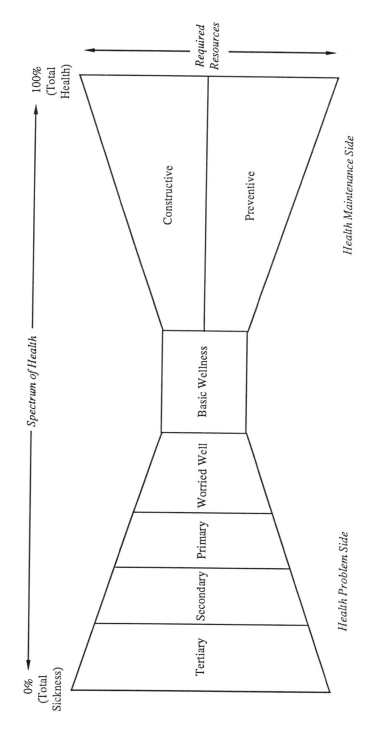

mous amount of resources. In areas toward the middle of the diagram, a relatively large move to the right can be made with relatively less expenditure of resources. Then, as we progress into the right side of the diagram, increasingly large amounts of resources are once again required to approach "total health."

The real significance of this model is that, except for the tertiary care level at the left, the entire spectrum of health must be the concern of the ambulatory care provider. It is also significant that this includes the entire right side of the spectrum; thus, there are many "health related," as opposed to purely medical, dimensions to an ambulatory care program. A truism in the ambulatory care setting is that our patients come to us with problems that are not always strictly medical. The many components of a human being's life are all interrelated in complex fashion; the patients themselves may not be aware whether their problems are actually physical, social, or psychological—or a combination of these factors. Ambulatory care, therefore, must by its very nature assume a truly "whole person" approach to care.

For all of these reasons, Quality Assurance in ambulatory care is extraordinarily complex. The task must, however, be undertaken—the stakes are simply too high not to do so.

Current Developmental Challenges in Quality Assurance

The field of Quality Assurance in health care is currently a fascinating place to be. Quality Assurance professionals are at last seeing concrete results from their efforts, and they are noticing the broader health care field taking increasing notice of *them*. Quality Assurance is becoming ever more energized, and much of this energy is being focused on continually improving the discipline itself; the result is that assessment technology is becoming increasingly visible, viable, and effective. In short, this is an exciting time to be involved in this developing field.

But while highly promising trends are being seen in several important areas, the work is far from complete. The following major issues represent areas of both past achievement and current challenge.

Physician Acceptance

The heart and soul of quality in a clinical organization must be the performance of the provider staff itself; therefore, physicians must be willing to publicly endorse and actively participate in ongoing Quality Assurance development and implementation. Historically, however, this has sometimes proven difficult. Walter McClure, president of the Center for Policy Studies, uses the term "provider divisiveness" for what has frequently occurred when physicians have been requested to participate in formal Quality Assurance activity. McClure asserts (1987): "'Provider divisiveness'—that's a polite word. . . that means what your colleagues do with a hatchet axe between your shoulder blades when you suggest that they might want to be measured (for quality). . . ."

Fortunately, we are seeing a decided change in this type of thinking; more and more physicians are viewing Quality Assurance as a real opportunity, rather than as a threat. Creative and committed physicians are emerging as national leaders in conceptual Quality Assurance development. The first challenge, then, is to continually build upon this growing nucleus, so that all providers are eventually convinced that Quality Assurance is undeniably worth the time, effort, and cost.

Many physicians continue to ask a legitimate question: "Will Quality Assurance really improve the health of my patients?" The most visible challenge here is, of course, to develop meaningful systems that ultimately *do* impact health status. A significant underlying challenge is to actively demonstrate a definitive cause-and-effect relationship between ongoing Quality Assurance and patient health.

Another necessary task is to develop peer review to the point at which it becomes a visibly constructive and well-accepted activity, rather than one that too often generates hard feelings among the professional staff. (For our interpretation of "peer review," as well as for definitions of other terms in this book, please refer to the glossary displayed as Resource D.) Problems discovered through the peer assessment process must be handled professionally, discreetly, and (as specifically noted in the Quality Assurance plans of several of our study sites) confidentially. In addition, provider input must be an integral part of setting clinical criteria and standards that are demonstrably rational and professionally valid.

Organizational Acceptance

Especially in the ambulatory care setting, many centers performing Quality Assurance have traditionally done so primarily because it was required, most often for external accreditation. Relatively few ambulatory care organizations have historically been involved with formal assessment solely because it is inherently a good idea; as McClure suggests (1987), "It's easy to invent the Pill—what's hard is to convince the pope."

A growing number of ambulatory care organizations now realize, however, that Quality Assurance can have a substantial and positive impact on their overall programs. Ambulatory care Quality Assurance, although in many ways still in its infancy, is nevertheless light years ahead of where it was ten years ago; a primary reason is that more ambulatory care organizations now believe in the inherent value of the process and are making the commitment to develop strong programs for their own sake.

There is a whole complex of challenges for ambulatory care centers today in performing effective Quality Assurance.

Cost. The simple fact is that we don't have a commonly accepted notion of how much reliable Quality Assurance actually costs. In addition, it is difficult at best to quantify with any certainty the return on this unknown investment. Organizations are, therefore, sometimes reluctant to commit to a major proposition for which the bottom line is uncertain. It has been suggested (O'Leary, 1987, p. 3) that 1 percent of the total organizational budget should be spent on assessment—and this sounds like a lot of money. But can we honestly say that this is verifiably too much?

If an organization wishes to perform valid Quality Assurance, it must actively invest in the staff time required for data generation, as well as the expenses involved in the monitoring and evaluation process itself. The organization can minimize these costs by ensuring that the bulk of the work is clerical in nature (calling upon expensive professional time only to address issues that professionals alone can handle), that data being collected continue to be required or useful, and that special studies are critically appraised whenever their costs appear excessive. But no matter how efficient Quality Assurance may become, it will still be a generator of expense. And there is yet another, more indirect, cost involved—the expense of actually improving quality once a problem is found through assessment.

Therefore, the current cost-related challenge is to develop a true understanding both of the real total costs of Quality Assurance and of its "return on investment." In essence, one of the tasks facing the field is to require of itself what it demands of organizations—the development of generally accepted standards for its own operation.

Comprehensiveness. To a large degree, Quality Assurance programs today are still not sufficiently comprehensive; many remain in the rudimentary stage at which the program looks at a few specific issues but decidedly not at the total picture. It is important to monitor all relevant performance, including both specific clinical issues and important administrative functions which enable the provision of clinical care. The challenge here is to develop a total monitoring and evaluation program that is truly an ongoing, structured review of the entire operation, especially as it affects clinical care.

Appropriate Processes. A number of ambulatory care centers remain confused about what "monitoring and evaluation" really includes. Some organizations still essentially address medical care evaluation studies, while others perform what are really problem-finding exercises. Thus, we are in some ways still rooted in Quality Assurance's past. Our challenge in this area is to continue development of a full and universal understanding of true assessment and its component processes.

Real Organizational Commitment. A fundamental problem in some organizations is still the lack of real top-level commitment to, and "clout" for, the assessment program. Quality Assurance committees can spin their wheels almost endlessly, doing what seems to be their job, but if Quality Assurance is not functionally a top priority of the organization, the program simply cannot work with best effect. There must be constant reinforcement that the needs of Quality Assurance *will* be met and that identified problems *will* be solved. The challenge is to fully convince governing bodies and top management once and for all that Quality Assurance is inherently valuable, that the program's results will indeed foster the organizational mission, and that there must be sufficient and clear organizational commitment if the assessment program is to function as intended.

National Leadership

During the 1970s, there was for all practical purposes no strong, commonly accepted national leadership in the Quality Assurance field, especially in the ambulatory care setting. However, in the last decade several organizations (including those noted previously) have begun to step forward to provide real leadership. Unfortunately, the directions taken by these groups are not always fully consistent, with the result that it is sometimes easy to be confused by what the national leaders seem to be telling us.

Even within what is generally regarded as one of the foremost organizations addressing Quality Assurance today, JCAHO, the ground rules seem to have changed several times in recent years. At the very least, significant changes in terminology may have muddied the water for some centers undertaking Quality Assurance as these changes were occurring.

Therefore, another major challenge is for the national leadership to forge a real consensus, then to lead the rest of us, step by logical step, toward truly effective programs based on this consensus. Additionally, these steps should be grounded in commonly accepted terminologies and definitions.

Development of Common Indicators and Standards

The lexicon continues to be volatile; but whatever terms we employ, it remains fundamental that a specific determination must be made regarding those factors that truly seem to affect the health of our patients. As a practical matter, assessment is chaotic until we agree on what we should be routinely monitoring and evaluating, and on what our performance should be in these areas.

Lack of common indicators of quality and generally accepted standards of care is still a pervasive problem in Quality Assurance. One result is that we have largely relegated our assessment programs to the structure and process realms, and we are only just beginning to talk with any real specificity about measures of outcome.

The simple fact is that many ambulatory care organizations still have not explicitly and prospectively defined their own most important issues and expectations. This is a critical problem. Quality Assurance committees cannot adequately monitor and evaluate the performance of their organizations until these issues and expectations have been clearly defined. Defining and developing clinically oriented indicators and standards, especially as they relate to outcomes, is an extraordinarily difficult task; our present challenge is to undertake the process in earnest.

Quality Management

One of the most important goals of Quality Assurance is to ultimately enable an organization to actively *manage* the quality of the care it provides; at present, however, relatively little activity of this nature has been successfully accomplished. One fundamental reason is that we simply have not yet developed effective and widely accepted methods of measuring (that is, quantifying) quality levels within our centers. The AmbuQual Quality Assurance program, described later in this book, is a positive step, but much remains to be done.

The primary challenge, then, is to develop systems that will routinely generate the necessary quantitative data to enable us to actually manage, and not just superficially address, quality.

Summary

In an era of cost containment and competition, we clearly have some powerful mandates for ensuring that a true regard for quality remains paramount. In the words of Robert Cunningham (1984), a contributing editor of *Hospitals* magazine, "The *real* threat to my grandchildren and their children, it seems to me, is not in the forms and finances (of health care)...but in the underlying motivation that moves the system. . . . There can be only one overarching value for the sake of which everything else is done, and that has to be patient access and patient care."

Chapter 2

Developing a Framework
for Quality Assurance

On the other hand, if Quality is subjective, existing only
in the observer, then this Quality that you make so much
of is just a fancy name for whatever you like.
> — Robert M. Pirsig, *Zen and*
> *the Art of Motorcycle*
> *Maintenance*

The forces of cost and quality are potentially on a collision
course. Due largely to financial considerations, the very foundations of what most people think of as quality in health care are
threatened. That is the bad news. The good news is that defend-
ing the right to continue to deliver quality care is precisely the
function addressed by a strong Quality Assurance system. There
are, however, some potential difficulties to be encountered along
the way.

Confounding Factors

Both in conception and implementation, Quality Assurance can become complex, for a number of reasons.

***Difficulties in Structuring and Integrating the Quality Assurance
Function.*** A number of otherwise excellent ambulatory care
centers have encountered difficulty because they have responded to the Quality Assurance initiative by simply appoint-
ing a Quality Assurance committee and instructing this new
entity to "start doing Quality Assurance." These committees

have then too often been left to flounder, with no specific guidance on exactly how to accomplish this task. The committees sometimes discover a scarcity of available organizational capacity and resources (including time) to perform true quality assessment; a common sentiment is, "We already have more than enough to do just taking care of our patients."

This is symptomatic of what might be termed the "tack-on phenomenon," in which a Quality Assurance function is merely tacked on to an existing organizational structure with little thought and less direction. This can easily lead to justifiable complaints from all quarters.

A General Uncertainty Regarding Terminology. Each field has its own set of terms; such a common language functions as a sort of working shorthand for persons working in the field. Problems arise, however, when this terminology is in continual flux; unfortunately, such has been the recent history in Quality Assurance. For example, the term "monitor" is often employed differently by different organizations, and it is sometimes used interchangeably with other words (such as "indicator") within the same organization. Terms such as "aspect of care" and "threshold" can enter (and sometimes exit) the common language seemingly overnight, or can permutate to mean something new just as quickly. Both an overly fluid terminology and a changing conceptual base can easily confound implementation of a viable assessment program. In this book, we shall use what we believe are now becoming reasonably standard terms. (As an aid to the use of these terms, we have included a glossary as Resource D.)

The Range of Initial Choices That Must Be Made. Should we be trying to assess the structure of our organization, the process of care delivery, or the actual outcome of care? If we choose outcome, should we focus on initial outcomes (such as complications of various procedures), long-term outcomes (the ultimate effects on health), or both? Should we focus on purely clinical matters, or do we also need to look at administrative issues as well? Do we create special data-gathering systems, or simply use what already exists?

The effect of these confounding factors can be real confusion for a new or developing Quality Assurance program. What one Quality Assurance coordinator (Wildman, 1988, p. 18) has stated regarding a specific system can probably be applied to the overall field of Quality Assurance at present: "[The] lack of definitive descriptions of the terminology and process has left many of those responsible for conducting quality assurance activities to struggle. . . . The result has often been confusion and uncertainty. . . ."

Even in the best of existing programs, this can be a problem. As Inge Winer, one of the Quality Assurance professionals we interviewed, stated, "We often feel as if we have to invent the wheel. What's needed is more specific help for developing programs, and more active interface with other Quality Assurance professionals." Our own AmbuQual program, the highly structured ambulatory care Quality Assurance system profiled later in this book, was in large part a response to our own need for a system to operationalize Quality Assurance as concretely as possible.

What seems to be called for, then, is a conceptual model that can be commonly accepted and can generate appropriate standard terminology. It should be specific enough to provide concrete guidance on how to assess quality, what to assess, and what to do with the resulting evaluative information; it should also be general enough to be flexible, so that unique organizational needs can be addressed.

Our model must meet another requirement as well. There are three progressive stages through which Quality Assurance must move if maximum benefit is to be derived:

- *monitoring and assessing* quality,
- actively *measuring* quality, and
- *managing* quality.

As a practical matter, most of what is being done currently centers on the first stage; while some initial work is beginning to measure quality, very little as yet is being done to actually manage quality. Nevertheless, our proposed Quality Assurance model should lend itself to any of these three stages, and it should be structured such that an organization may make the transition with relative ease from one stage to the next.

Happily, such a model can easily be constructed on foundations that already exist. This model is largely based on the conceptual framework being promoted by what we believe will become the accepted national leader in Quality Assurance, the Joint Commission. It is also the basic model being used by the five highly functional Quality Assurance programs we visited in researching this book (as noted in the Preface and in Chapter Three). We will outline this generic model as a usable structure for program development, after first addressing three basic processes underpinning Quality Assurance implementation; the chapters in Part Two will then build on the model's progressive steps, using examples from our five study sites as illustration.

Three Basic Quality Assurance Tasks

The Quality Assurance philosophy must be woven into the basic fabric of the entire organization. Although Quality Assurance is a specific program, it cannot be effective unless the entire organization—from the governing body on down—understands and accepts basic Quality Assurance concepts and is committed to making assessment really work. Therefore, Quality Assurance must be both a "top-down" and "bottom-up" phenomenon. Accordingly, the following tasks should be addressed early, to ensure that the program ultimately developed will most effectively graft itself onto the organization.

Establish the Mission First. This is the top-down portion of the overall approach. Quality Assurance must begin with the governing body, since this group is ultimately responsible for the quality of care provided by the organization. The governing body should be sure that the mission statement of the organization contains a requirement for systematic activity that routinely assures quality; it must also actively nurture this activity.

Quality Assurance programs that do not enjoy active top-down involvement are both shallow and endangered. The top level of the organization should actively commission the program, buy into the inherent value of Quality Assurance, and direct the total organization to perform Quality Assurance on its behalf. Assessment will then become a fundamental component of the organization, rather than a tack-on phenomenon.

The governing body should establish the specific purpose of the Quality Assurance program, consistent with the mission of the organization itself. There are many potential purposes, such as public accountability, general risk management, third-party accountability, and external accreditation. The governing body should also specify clear objectives for the Quality Assurance program (usually as stated in a Quality Assurance plan); since these will be felt throughout the organization, the governing body should play a key role in their establishment.

The point here is simply that commissioning the program, as well as specifying its purpose and program objectives, is the role of the governing body, not of the Quality Assurance committee or the organization's management. The solid foundation thus built will support the Quality Assurance program over the long haul.

Develop the Quality Related Structures of the Organization Before Writing the Quality Assurance Plan or Establishing the Quality Assurance Committee. Developing these structures is the bottom-up portion of a total approach to Quality Assurance, and it is the responsibility of administration. Quality Assurance will be functionally anemic unless the organization has strong quality related activities already in place as candidates for evaluation. Thus, the task is to ensure that these quality related components are in good shape.

Every ambulatory care organization probably already has a significant number of quality related activities occurring continually. These are generally of three types: quality control activities, quality improvement activities, and quality patient care activities.

It is likely that every organization in the business of delivering ambulatory care routinely processes lab unknowns; this is quality control. Generic quality control consists of activities designed to prevent unwanted change. Other examples include job descriptions, performance evaluations, repeated provider credentialing processes, policies and procedures, patient satisfaction studies, and chart audits. The sum of all such activities can be thought of as the "quality floor" for the organization.

Quality improvement activities have the objective of creating positive change. In-service training, continuing education, and incentive systems are some examples. Revising outdated job descriptions or modifying existing policies and procedures can also create positive change. The totality of these activities can be thought of as the "quality staircase" for the organization.

Quality patient care activities include everything that occurs in the critical interface between provider and patient. Quality patient care activities address the basic health care mandates of effectiveness, efficiency, appropriateness, acceptability, and accessibility; thus, the strength of the medical staff itself is critical here. The "quality floor" and the "quality staircase" together form the structure upon which this ongoing quality patient care is built.

Note that these are quality *related* activities, not full-blown Quality Assurance; however, each must be firmly in place before the assessment program can be fully developed. The primary role of Quality Assurance, then, is to monitor these activities regularly, to ensure that they are truly functional and are actively contributing to the health of the patient.

Develop the Overall Quality Assurance Program. So what, then, *is* Quality Assurance? Simply put, it is a self-contained oversight program to assure that all needed quality related activities are present and are optimally effective; that the results of ongoing quality related activity are positive; and that these results are appropriately and positively communicated, understood, and facilitated.

Quality Assurance routinely provides a structured and comprehensive assessment of the total ambulatory care program and a mechanism for solving problems it identifies. The analogy of renal dialysis may be helpful in visualizing this concept. The ongoing flow of quality related activity within the body of the organization is continually passed through the filter of the Quality Assurance process. Any "impurities" are corrected and returned to the organizational body in an improved state, while quality related activities displaying no problems return to the stream unaltered.

We have now ensured the top-down/bottom-up involvement of both the policy-making and operational components of the organization, and we have added a specific process known as Quality Assurance to oversee and facilitate all quality related activities within the ambulatory care center. With these basics firmly in place, we turn our attention to a specific model for the Quality Assurance process itself.

A Generic Model for Quality Assurance

The model below, based on that promoted by JCAHO, is designed to provide a step-by-step methodology for development and implementation of a Quality Assurance program that is systematic, ongoing, comprehensive, and integrated. The resulting system will ensure that Quality Assurance involves all appropriate persons; that evaluation is based on collection of specified data; and that identified problems are actively addressed, solved, and continually monitored. Through this model, programs at all levels should find useful guidance. It can assist both in uncovering patterns of care that might need improvement and in focusing on individual cases that could lead to identification of specific correctable problems.

Quality Assurance as a Two-Phase Process. The model also addresses the two-phase nature of Quality Assurance: looking for potential problems or opportunities for improvement, and assuring solutions to those problems and activating identified opportunities. These two phases are commonly referred to as "monitoring and evaluation" and "problem resolution."

The current conceptual framework for Quality Assurance is that of a systematic monitoring and evaluation of the entire clinical care program provided by an ambulatory care organization. The term "monitoring" connotes actively tracking something routinely; this can mean once a day, once a week, once a month, or even once a year, depending on the perceived significance of the area. Rather than a program comprising essentially random studies, there should be a systematic plan for reviewing all important elements of the clinical program (as well as elements of the administrative program that have an impact on clinical care) on a prescheduled basis.

Evaluation of the monitored areas is the next task. Simply stated, to evaluate means to make some sort of judgment. In a health care Quality Assurance setting, this judgment is based on predetermined, clinically valid criteria and related standards — that is, those that would make sense to external providers and have consensus approval from the organization itself. Some person or group must then analyze data regarding performance against these criteria and standards, in order to judge that performance.

If the evaluation indicates that there are no problems, then all is well. If, on the other hand, evaluation indicates potential problems, then a designated person or group should take appropriate problem-solving action (including future re-evaluation, to ensure that the situation, once changed, remains changed for the better). Even if no obvious problems exist, this second phase of Quality Assurance can assure the organization that it continually capitalizes on identified opportunities to improve its ambulatory care program. These activities in combination foster the continuous improvement in performance that is the hallmark of an effective Quality Assurance system.

The combined results of these two fundamental phases of Quality Assurance must then become part of an ongoing permanent record. There should be a recognized "trail" of minimum but appropriate documentation from the outset — from the initial commissioning of the program by the governing body, to the development of the Quality Assurance plan, to the documented results of monitoring and evaluation activities, through the tracking of all problems to final resolution.

The Nine-Step Model. Let us now look at the specific steps for our model of Quality Assurance development. Part Two of this book will provide specific examples of each; in addition, Exhibit 1 shows how our own program in Indianapolis has addressed each of the nine steps.

> *Step One:* Determine the *focus of responsibility* of organizational Quality Assurance activity.
>
> *Step Two:* Determine the *scope of services* being generated by the organization.
>
> *Step Three:* Select *significant aspects of care* for the organization to track routinely.
>
> *Step Four:* Choose *specific indicators of quality* to monitor; these indicators should relate directly to the important aspects of care that have been chosen.
>
> *Step Five:* Develop *criteria* regarding performance for the selected indicators of quality and establish related *standards* for measuring performance.
>
> *Step Six:* Routinely and systematically *monitor and evaluate* the chosen indicators of quality, through the collection and analysis of appropriate performance data.
>
> *Step Seven:* Take appropriate *problem resolution action* when the organization's performance standard has not been met, as identified through the monitoring and evaluation process. This can take the form of either more intensive evaluation activity (generally by professional personnel) or immediate assignment of action to correct an evident problem or to pursue a clear opportunity for improvement.
>
> *Step Eight: Track resulting corrective actions or improvements,* to be sure they are continually effective.
>
> *Step Nine: Create a permanent record* of all Quality Assurance activities, ensuring that all relevant information is *fully integrated* into the organization.

Specific Terminology Considerations. Several key terms in the foregoing model may be unfamiliar; the most important of these are probably "aspects of care" and "indicators of quality." In fact, these terms are rapidly becoming commonplace in

Exhibit 1. Implementing the Nine-Step Model: An Example.

Step One: "Determine Focus of Responsibility." Assigned multidisciplinary Quality
   Assurance committee, which reports to executive director and governing body.
Step Two: "Determine Scope of Services." "Inventoried" clinical services and administrative enabling functions within organization, from procedures lists, cata-
   logues of formal protocols, administrative policies/procedures manuals, medical record system. Synthesized services/management functions into ten general
   "parameters of care" (see Chapter Nine).
Step Three: "Select Important 'Aspects of Care.'" Selected most important clinical
   services and administrative functions for each parameter of care. *Example:*
   Aspect = "Medical Records Policies" (within "Medical Records System"
   parameter).
Step Four: "Choose Specific 'Indicators of Quality' Relating to Selected Aspects of Care."
   Chose measurable facets of performance (within selected aspects) that would
   reasonably indicate quality. *Example:* Indicator = "Timeliness of Medical Records Entry" (within "Medical Records Policies" aspect).
Step Five: "Develop Criteria and Standards for Chosen Indicators." Assigned organizationally generated criteria for all indicators; developed, with participation of
   all top-level clinical/administrative directors, consensus standards for these
   criteria. *Example:* Criterion = "All medical records entries must be made within
   forty-eight hours of clinical activity." Related Standard = "No more than 20
   percent deficiency rate."
*Step Six: "Routinely Monitor Selected Indicators and Evaluate Quality of Each (Through
   Collection/Analysis of Performance Data)."* Developed prospective ongoing schedule of monitoring, by specific indicators. Routinely collected needed data
   through a "data source" specified for each indicator. Comparison of resulting
   data against selected criteria/standards performed at monthly Quality Assurance committee meetings. *Example:* Collected data on timeliness of medical
   records entry via ongoing procedural audit; when indicator scheduled for
   review, Quality Assurance committee analyzed audit results and compared
   against standard.
Step Seven: "Take Problem Resolution Action When Standards Are Not Met." Assigned
   action, whenever needed, to appropriate and prospectively specified managers. *Example:* If the deficiency rate for timeliness of medical records entry was
   greater than 20 percent, committee would assign corrective action to the
   medical director.
Step Eight: "Track Resulting Corrective Actions." Assigned specified deadlines for
   corrective action; at deadline, rescored indicator and followed up as needed.
   Example: If medical records timeliness problems were not solved by deadline (as
   verified by new comparison of performance data with standard), corrective
   action memo forwarded by committee to executive director; if still not solved
   by second deadline, committee would send problem to governing body.
*Step Nine: "Create a Permanent Record, and Integrate the Information into the Organiza-
   tion."* Quality Assurance committee meeting minutes routinely distributed
   throughout the organization (to all staff and governing body members); written
   documentation of all corrective action assignments, reevaluations, and subsequent action accomplished via a "quality improvement plan" (QIP), as noted in
   Chapter Nine.

Source: Community Health Network, Inc., Indianapolis.

discussions of Quality Assurance; unfortunately, many programs either are not aware of the functional definitions of these terms or tend to use them interchangeably.

Significant aspects of care are simply the organization's selection of the most important items from its scope of services inventory, as determined in Step Two of the model; these should include those services, procedures, or presenting conditions that are "high-volume, high-risk, or problem-prone" (Joint Commission on Accreditation of Healthcare Organizations, 1988, p. 6).

An indicator of quality within any given aspect of care, then, is a variable relating to the structure, process, or outcome of that aspect (as further explained later) that can be defined and measured through appropriate data collection; it should also have clear relevance to the quality of the aspect under scrutiny. Simply stated, an indicator is what is reviewed through the routine monitoring and evaluation process described above.

Thus, an indicator is a functional subset of an aspect. In practice, this means that while no specific indicator should relate directly to more than one aspect, an aspect may contain more than one indicator. For example, if the organization agrees that "clinical information availability" is an important aspect of the care it provides, it might decide that an indicator of quality is "patients seen without a record," with a procedural chart audit as the data source. An additional indicator for the same aspect might be the "timeliness" of routine entry of clinical information into the medical record.

We believe that these terms will grow in importance and acceptance, ultimately becoming a standard part of the lexicon. It will thus be important for organizations to specifically and prospectively define both their important aspects of care and associated indicators of quality, as well as the specific relationships among them.

Before leaving our discussion of specific terminology, we must also address our conscious avoidance of the relatively new term "thresholds." This is primarily a Joint Commission term; unfortunately, it has the potential to cause confusion. The full term is "thresholds for evaluation," reflecting the belief that "to conclude that there is a problem requires intensive evaluation of the care provided" (Joint Commission on Accreditation of Healthcare Organizations, 1988, p. 7). We believe that this is largely intended to address provider concern that a clinical indicator cannot by itself determine if good care has been delivered; JCAHO's desire is to promote the idea that indicators serve mainly as "screens" for potential problems.

In fact, clinical practice must always rely ultimately on the day-to-day judgments made by providers, and there will always be cases in which, for valid reasons, all elements of an established protocol are not followed. Partly with this in mind, JCAHO has generated a model that has one more step than our own. This falls immediately after the analysis of appropriate data (Step Six in our model), and it requires that the organization "evaluate care when the thresholds are reached" (Joint Commission on Accreditation of Healthcare Organizations, 1988, p. 4). In essence, this is a mandatory second evaluation. Under JCAHO's model, a determination that a problem exists is not finally made until the data are first found to be below the assigned "threshold," and subsequent additional in-depth evaluation is accomplished.

We believe, however, that there are times when initial evaluation alone indicates a clear problem. We also believe that justifiable deviations from standard clinical practice can be just as easily accommodated within a simpler model. We therefore rely on the more common concept of "standards," and we avoid the potentially confusing new term "thresholds."

Other Suggestions on Monitoring. Now that we have clarified some related terminology, it is appropriate to touch upon two additional notions that are important to the two-phase nature of Quality Assurance described above.

First, an organization should prospectively determine the desired frequency of monitoring. An initial judgment must be made regarding the significance of the aspects of care selected for monitoring; this decision will then largely dictate how frequently these areas should be evaluated. Inherent in the decision must be a consideration of the consequences of problems within the aspect whose indicators are being evaluated. Generally, if it is very likely that a problem within the aspect could have a significant impact on the health of the patient, then relatively frequent review of most or all of the related indicators is probably called for. If, however, there is a less serious potential impact, then the organization might well decide to review some or all of these indicators less frequently. Since both data gathering and active evaluation can be time consuming and costly, this notion is clearly important. Do not squander precious resources in overly frequent monitoring of relatively less important issues.

Once monitoring frequency has been decided, it is easy to develop a schedule for ensuring that all necessary reviews occur as desired. A monitoring and evaluation schedule can be developed for an entire year in advance, thereby setting up a clear road map for the Quality Assurance committee. This frees the committee to grapple with the more important task of actually *performing* the needed monitoring and evaluation activity.

Second, the organization must monitor the monitoring. While this may initially sound like so much double-talk, it is nevertheless vital to the long-term success of a Quality Assurance program. Once monitoring has been undertaken, the organization must be certain that such activity is actually occurring on a routine basis, and that a functional system exists by which problems are actively resolved and opportunities for improvements are specifically pursued. This is accomplished partly through the selection of appropriate instruments to document and report ongoing Quality Assurance activity, and partly through the annual Quality Assurance program review that should be performed.

In this chapter we have addressed both the basic concepts that undergird quality assessment and a specific nine-step model that can serve as a practical, step-by-step guide to the development of a solid Quality Assurance program. This model can help bring a sense of order to a sometimes seemingly chaotic field. Bruce Biller, Quality Assurance committee chairperson at one of our five study sites, when asked what suggestions he would make to other programs, stated emphatically,

"Be systematic: Organize, organize, organize!" The beauty of our model is that it provides a ready-made framework for just that.

A first-rate Quality Assurance program cannot, however, develop overnight; like anything worthwhile, it will take time. Magda Cockerline, director of nursing at another of our study sites, was asked what she thought was needed to ensure an effective program. Her reply: "Seeds and water. . .seeds and water." Our nine-step model will provide the necessary seeds; time, patience, and commitment will provide the nurturing water.

Chapter 3

Quality Assurance Programs in Five Diverse Settings

Perhaps one could learn as much, or even more, about how to foster quality by also studying the occurrence and localization of superlative performance.
— Avedis Donabedian

Quality Assurance is being discussed, implemented, and refined in ambulatory care settings of all types. But while one can go to a fair number of sources to research health care Quality Assurance theory, it is still difficult to find much on how Quality Assurance systems actually function in specific ambulatory care settings.

This book intends to help remedy this situation. Most of the remaining chapters will deal with specific ways to implement the generic Quality Assurance model suggested in Chapter Two. We will be drawing from five specific case examples; these programs from across the country will help demonstrate functional Quality Assurance mechanisms in a variety of ambulatory care settings. (An explanation of our site selection process and detailed individual descriptions of each organization and its Quality Assurance program are given in Resource A.) Our intent throughout the rest of this book is to be descriptive rather than prescriptive. We believe that, as the old aphorism maintains, there is indeed "more than one way to skin a cat," and we feel confident that virtually any new or developing Quality Assurance program can find some helpful ideas for its own setting from among the variety of workable program examples presented throughout this book.

The Sites and Contact Persons

We have selected five case examples that are diverse yet
share some common themes in Quality Assurance development
and implementation. They represent many intersecting dynamics with regard to organizational and Quality Assurance program structure, size, function, program complexity, and so
forth. The sites, alphabetically by city, are as follows:

1. (Atlanta, Georgia) Southeastern Health Services, a propri-
    etary group practice;
2. (Cambridge, Massachusetts) The MIT Medical Department,
    an integrated system at the Massachusetts Institute of Tech-
    nology with major prepaid /HMO involvement;
3. (Chicago, Illinois) The University of Chicago Hospitals, a
    major university-affiliated health complex;
4. (Fremont, California) Washington Outpatient Surgery Cen-
    ter, a hospital-affiliated ambulatory surgery facility; and
5. (Indianapolis, Indiana) Community Health Network, Inc., a
    system of three community health centers managed by a
    major urban hospital, with a primary mission of indigent
    care. (This system, more commonly known as "HealthNet," is
    our own organization.)

We should note that in both the following pages and
Resource A we describe these programs largely as they existed
when we visited them. However, since no system of any type can
remain static and still thrive, these five programs will look at
least somewhat different when this book is read than they did
when we wrote about them. Such is the nature of publishing; it is
also, fortunately, the nature of organizational development and
improvement. These systems, no matter what may have changed
since, were uniformly effective as described throughout this
book.

At each of these five sites, we spoke at length to one or
more persons who either were integral to Quality Assurance
program development or were instrumental in the ongoing
operation of the existing system, as follows:

1. In Atlanta, we met with Frank Houser and Mary Driscoll. Houser is president, board chairperson, and medical director of Southeastern Health Services; he is also chairperson of the Quality Assurance committee. Driscoll is director of quality control for the organization.
2. Our contacts in Cambridge were Bruce Biller and Rochelle Alexander. Biller functions as chairperson of the Quality Assurance committee, while Alexander is the Quality Assurance coordinator for the MIT Medical Department.
3. At The University of Chicago Hospitals, we spoke with Inge Winer, a social worker who is the Quality Assurance coordinator for this program.
4. In Fremont, we interviewed Magda Cockerline, the director of nursing for Washington Outpatient Surgery Center and a major participant in Quality Assurance program development for the facility.
5. At Community Health Network, of course, we relied primarily on our own experience. In addition, we consulted Jane Miller, the Quality Assurance coordinator for our system.

Processes, Observations, and General Results

To help standardize our interviews, we developed a six-page interview questionnaire that was sent to each site prior to our visit; the questions addressed each of the major steps in our generic Quality Assurance model (shown in Chapter Two), as well as such issues as the level of organizational acceptance of Quality Assurance activities, perceived benefits and drawbacks of Quality Assurance within the organization, and so forth.

The results of our visits quite frankly surprised us. Although we had expected diversity among these programs, we had not expected the degree of diversity we found. While each Quality Assurance system is clearly effective, these five sites use a range of differing approaches. Some, for instance, focus on structure and process, some mainly on outcome; some use one set of terms, some another; some allow the Quality Assurance committee to help solve problems, while others do not; and so on.

Furthermore, our initial anticipation had been that visible differences among these sites would primarily reflect variations in the types of organizations themselves; thus, for example, we anticipated different approaches to Quality Assurance at the ambulatory surgery site and the community health centers, springing primarily from the disparate functions of these distinct settings. However, as we sorted through the mountains of information afforded us by our interviews, it became evident that organizational type by itself could not, at least from these five examples, cause the programmatic differences we noted. Even though some observed differences could indeed be explained by setting, it began to appear that a complex of forces other than organizational function primarily motivated these variances.

Factors Affecting Program Differences. After lengthy consideration of the major programmatic variations, we offer four main factors that we believe help to account for most of these differences:

1. *Size* of the overall organization;
2. *Complexity* of the parent organization, and the accompanying complexity of the Quality Assurance program structure;
3. *Staff interrelationships* within the overall organization (often resulting largely from the size or complexity of the parent entity); and
4. The *management style, personality, and philosophy* of Quality Assurance developers and implementers. (The Quality Assurance systems in several of the sites we visited bore the clear stamp of one or two key persons in the organization.)

Various presentations of these four factors appear in each of the programs. Consequently, each looks different in some visible ways from all of the others but still hews to the basic concepts found in the generic Quality Assurance model described in the preceding chapter. The key, of course, is once again that no single format need be adhered to in order to effectively promote valid Quality Assurance. All of these programs, while they sometimes differ significantly in forms, methods, or underlying approaches to Quality Assurance, nevertheless have at least one overriding point of commonality—each is highly effective within its own setting; while they may all take different roads, they all get to Rome. Thus, while each program can teach something to, and learn something from, each of the others, all work effectively to continually "notch up" the quality of care provided to patients within their own specific settings. As Biller from MIT says of his program, "We're quite happy with what we have—it works for us."

The Contexts: Specific Organizational and Programmatic Variables. During our analysis, it also became clear that we were observing essentially a spectrum of important Quality Assurance variables within the ambulatory care environment, including the following:

1.   From relatively simple Quality Assurance frameworks to complex and highly refined structures;
2.   From stable constructs to those in varying degrees of transition;
3.   From largely decentralized Quality Assurance functions to those that were more consciously centralized;
4.   From relatively small parent organizations to those that were quite large;
5.   From primarily subjective Quality Assurance systems to those that were (to varying degrees) objective; and
6.   From programs mostly retrospective in their assessment activity to those more nearly concurrent.

In sum, there were decidedly no carbon copies among these programs.

Common Ground. It should be stated in the same breath, however, that there were in fact major points of commonality among these programs. A list of the most important patches of common ground would include the following:

1. All worked in some fashion from the general to the specific; that is, regardless of terminology, functional "aspects of care" generated particular "indicators of quality."
2. All involved some level of criteria and standards against which organizational performance was measured.
3. All generated and actively used specified data sets for evaluation.
4. All pursued active problem solving based on noted deficiencies or opportunities to improve care, and all actively tracked the results of this problem-solving effort through some mechanism.
5. All enjoyed strong organizational support, flowing directly from the top of the organization and stated through a written Quality Assurance plan.
6. All performed an annual appraisal of the overall Quality Assurance program itself, making necessary modifications to both the assessment program structure or process and to specific aspects of care or indicators of quality.

Thus, while each of these ambulatory care organizations may interpret Quality Assurance principles in its own way or develop specific assessment structures to meet the needs of its particular environment, there are nonetheless some basic shared notions to which developing Quality Assurance programs can look for guidance. These are based in the general principles and specific development steps described in the previous chapter and developed in greater detail in the next part of this book.

Summary of Programs

We have selected five programs that suitably represent the major types of ambulatory care providers today. As evidence of their effectiveness, each of the sites has received accreditation from the Joint Commission on Accreditation of Healthcare Organizations.

Since these programs will serve as reference points and examples throughout the rest of this book, a brief overview of the distinguishing characteristics and strengths of each is presented below (and will be further detailed in following chapters). In addition, organization charts showing the relationship of each Quality Assurance program to its parent organization are displayed as Figures 2 through 8.

Southeastern Health Services (Atlanta) is a proprietary group practice (see Figure 2) whose Quality Assurance system is in transition from a relatively informal program to a more structured, integrated, and formalized one. An unusual degree of top-level support for the Quality Assurance program results from the fact that the chairperson of the Quality Assurance committee also chairs the organization's board, serves as the group's president, and acts as medical director of the proprietary corporation. A highly sophisticated patient satisfaction program, recently implemented, addresses the specific quality related issue of acceptability of care in detail. Additionally, the Quality Assurance structure includes and integrates the often separate functions of utilization review and risk management.

The MIT Medical Department (Cambridge), provider of a broad range of health services in a university setting, enjoys a significant proportion of health maintenance organization (HMO) business. Strong top-level Quality Assurance emphasis is provided by the medical director, who also serves as both the department head within the MIT structure and the chairperson of the executive committee of the department's medical staff (see Figures 3 and 4). The Quality Assurance program is basically decentralized, and the Quality Assurance committee chairperson strongly believes that the committee should not itself be involved in performing actual Quality Assurance functions for its individual organizational components (shown in Figure 5). The program lends itself to quick corrective action, and it is overtly positioned in a "zero defects" mode regarding specific clinical standards. It also generally maintains extremely high program performance, due in part to the inherent nature of a

Figure 2. Southeastern Health Services, Inc., Administrative Organizational Chart.

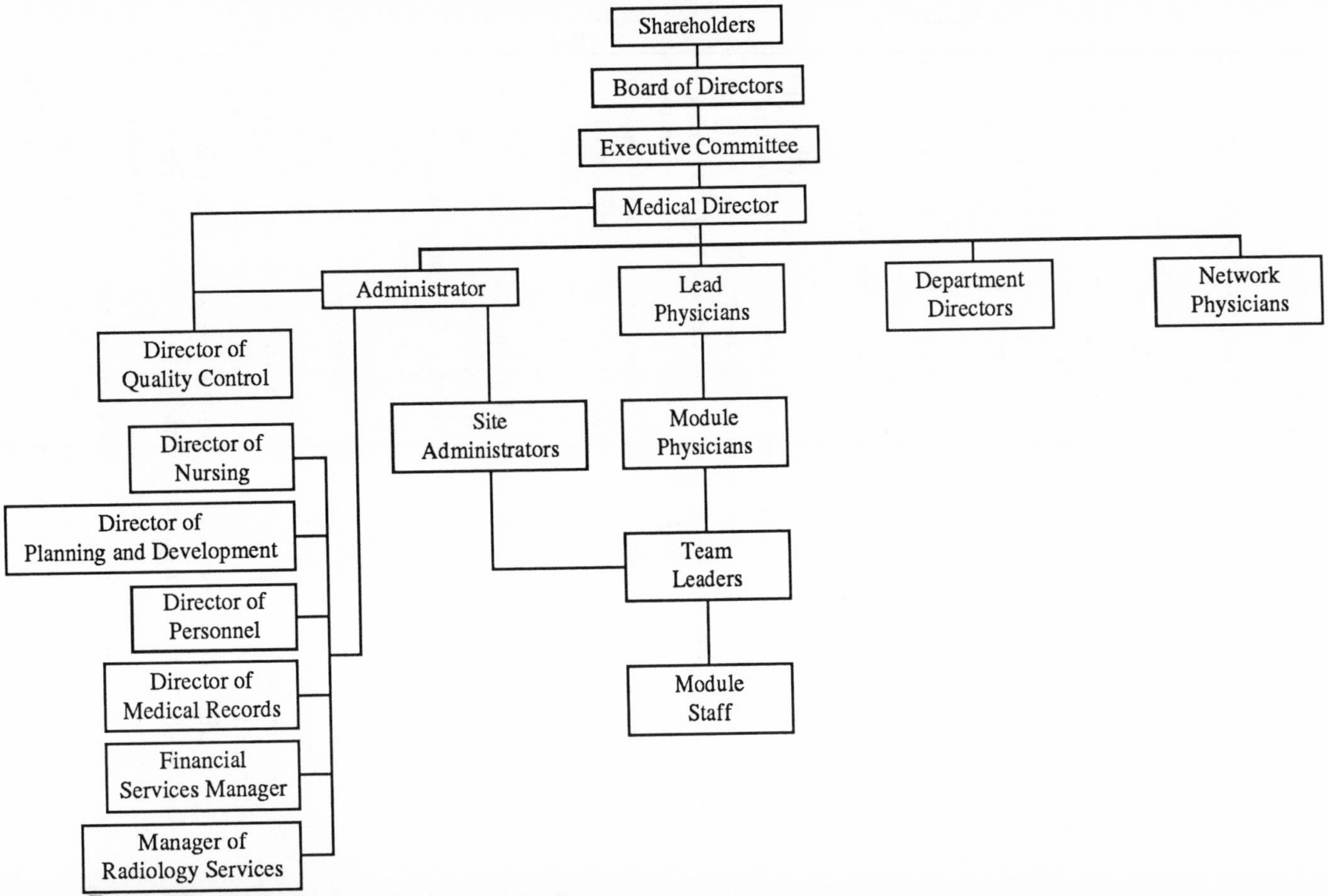

Shareholders

Board of Directors

Executive Committee

Medical Director

- Lead Physicians
  - Module Physicians
    - Team Leaders
      - Module Staff
- Department Directors
- Network Physicians

Administrator

- Site Administrators
- Director of Quality Control
- Director of Nursing
- Director of Planning and Development
- Director of Personnel
- Director of Medical Records
- Financial Services Manager
- Manager of Radiology Services

university staff and to the type of patients who use the department's services for their medical care. The program is also
among the most highly documented of those we studied.

The University of Chicago Hospitals program is the largest
and probably most complex of the five sites, due primarily to the
size and complexity of the overall hospitals system itself. The
organization's Quality Assurance plan is the most highly detailed, and outcome evaluation is heavily stressed throughout
the program. A strong degree of commitment from the highest
levels of the organization is evident. The system is moving toward a more integrated and prospectively oriented program,
which will focus on a broader array of indicators. An unspoken
"100 percent standard" exists by general consensus throughout
the system, due in part to the program's university base. Quality
Assurance is organizationally combined with utilization review.
For specific ambulatory care Quality Assurance within the overall hospitals framework, formal monitoring is performed during two one-week periods each year by every ambulatory care
clinic, using a standardized format. The Quality Assurance
organization is shown in Figure 6.

Washington Outpatient Surgery Center (Fremont) is the smallest and newest of the programs surveyed, and it has the least
complicated Quality Assurance system. The center functions as
a closely knit group in a "family" atmosphere, and this lends
itself to immediate problem solving and concurrent feedback.
The flow of Quality Assurance information and action is direct
and simple, data gathering is time consuming but well defined,
and the Quality Assurance process itself is largely decentralized.
All aspects and indicators are reviewed by the board once each
quarter within three areas of basically simultaneous day-to-day
activity: medical, nursing, and administrative (the business office and medical records functions); see Figure 7. The nature of
the organization allows Quality Assurance to be perhaps more
fully integrated into the actual daily routine of the staff than in
the other programs. Since the organization is itself only a few
years old and Quality Assurance activity began at virtually the
same time, the general concept of assessment enjoyed perhaps
more immediate and ready acceptance in this organization

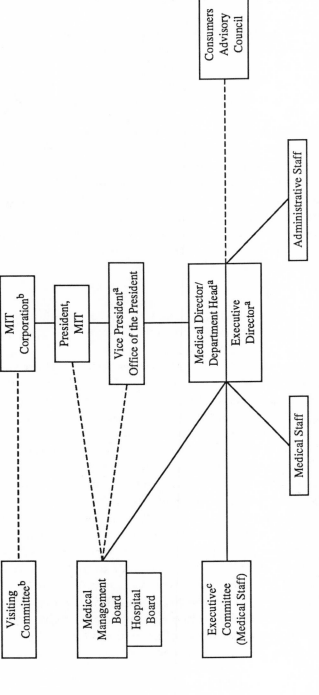

Figure 3. Massachusetts Institute of Technology: Governance of the Medical Department.

Consumers Advisory Council

Administrative Staff

MIT Corporation[b]

President, MIT

Vice President[a] Office of the President

Medical Director/ Department Head[a]

Executive Director[a]

Medical Staff

Visiting Committee[b]

Medical Management Board

Hospital Board

Executive[c] Committee (Medical Staff)

[a] Member of the Medical Management Board (MMB)
[b] Chairman of MMB is a Corporation Member and a member of the visiting committee
[c] Elected Representative of Medical Staff to MMB

Source: MIT Medical Department. Reprinted by permission.

Figure 4. MIT Medical Department Committees.

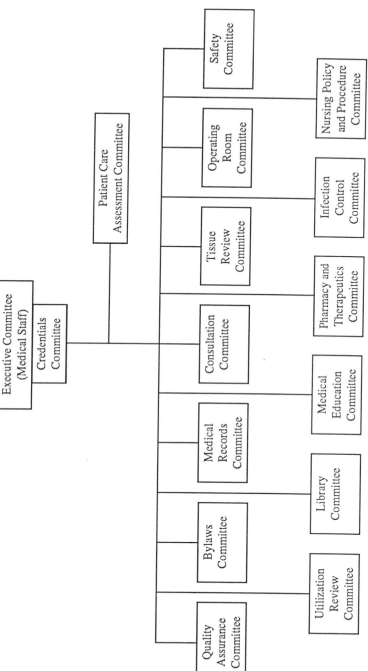

Source: MIT Medical Department. Reprinted by permission.

Figure 5. MIT Medical Department Quality Assurance Program Organizational Chart.

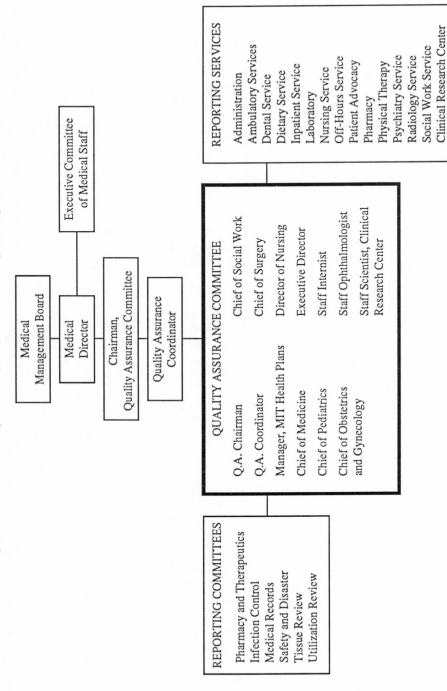

Medical
Management Board

Executive Committee
of Medical Staff

Medical
Director

Chairman,
Quality Assurance Committee

Quality Assurance
Coordinator

REPORTING COMMITTEES

Pharmacy and Therapeutics
Infection Control
Medical Records
Safety and Disaster
Tissue Review
Utilization Review

QUALITY ASSURANCE COMMITTEE

Q.A. Chairman
Q.A. Coordinator
Manager, MIT Health Plans
Chief of Medicine
Chief of Pediatrics
Chief of Obstetrics
and Gynecology

Chief of Social Work
Chief of Surgery
Director of Nursing
Executive Director
Staff Internist
Staff Ophthalmologist
Staff Scientist, Clinical
Research Center

REPORTING SERVICES

Administration
Ambulatory Services
Dental Service
Dietary Service
Inpatient Service
Laboratory
Nursing Service
Off-Hours Service
Patient Advocacy
Pharmacy
Physical Therapy
Psychiatry Service
Radiology Service
Social Work Service
Clinical Research Center

Figure 6. The University of Chicago Hospitals Quality Assurance Program Organizational Chart.

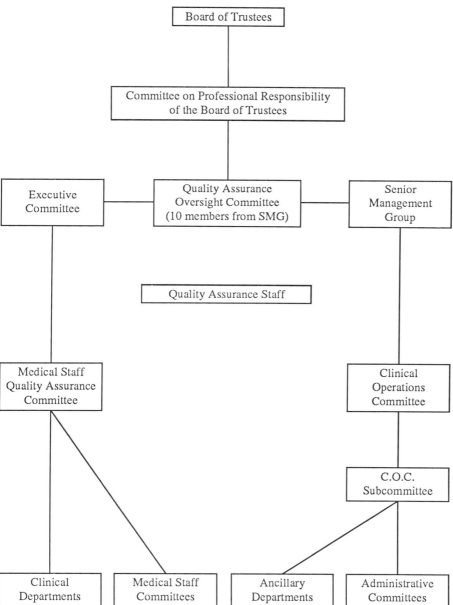

Source: Addendum 1 to "Quality Assurance Plan," Aug. 1987. Reprinted by permission.

than at any of the other sites researched. The current program, while basically stable, is also evolving.

Community Health Network, Inc. ("HealthNet") in Indianapolis (see Figure 8), whose Quality Assurance system is known as AmbuQual, has probably the most highly structured of the programs surveyed. It is also the only one that attempts to actively quantify the level of organizational quality over time, both for specific indicators and for the overall program. The AmbuQual system provides a highly specific role for a multi-disciplinary Quality Assurance committee, and it uses a formal instrument for identifying and assigning problems, specifying deadlines for resolution, formally closing the loop on final problem-solving activity, and reporting assessment results to the total organization. Within broad program areas known as "parameters of care," AmbuQual explicitly ties selected aspects of care to specified indicators of quality, as well as to prospectively generated criteria and standards specific to HealthNet. Since it is so highly standardized, this Quality Assurance system readily lends itself to total program computerization for monitoring, tracking, and quality value identification functions.

Summary

We have, we believe, chosen five sites that represent highly functional Quality Assurance technologies in a variety of representative ambulatory care settings. Each program can serve as a model in some way, and there is something in every one that can work for your program.

Figure 7. Washington Outpatient Surgery Center Quality Assurance Program Organizational Chart.

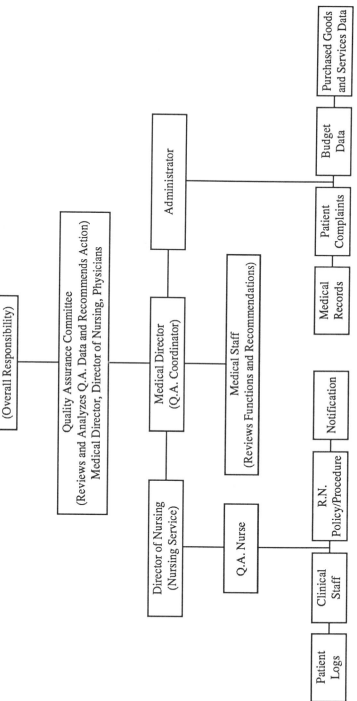

Source: Policy Manual, Book 1. Reprinted by permission.

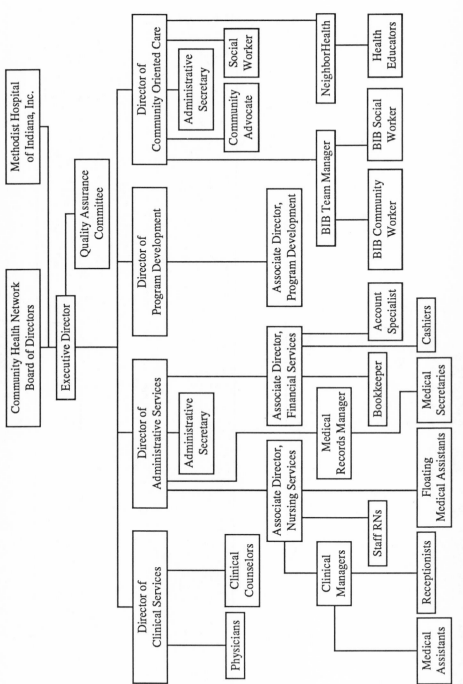

Figure 8. Community Health Network, Inc. Organizational Chart.

PART TWO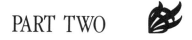

KEY COMPONENTS
IN DEVELOPING
A SUCCESSFUL
QUALITY ASSURANCE PROGRAM

Chapter 4

Defining the Aims
of Quality Assurance

The health of the people is really the foundation upon which all their happiness and their powers as a state depend.

— Benjamin Disraeli

For most professionals in ambulatory care, "mediocrity" is a four-letter word. All of the people who developed and helped implement our five studied programs would instinctively agree with an article (Johnson, 1987, p. 1) that described what is really one of the ultimate aims of Quality Assurance, the avoidance of mediocrity; this article asserted, "Settle for second-rate long enough, and eventually you won't recognize excellence when you see it. You'll forget that anything else is possible, and what's worse — you may not care."

The battle against mediocrity in medicine has many facets. Palmer proposes five major reasons for the emergence of formal Quality Assurance in health care:

- Some effective investigations and treatments are available: they should be provided to appropriate patients.
- Most investigations and treatments have dangerous side effects: they should be avoided for inappropriate patients.
- New investigations and treatments increase the cost of health care: they should be avoided for inappropriate patients.
- Prevention and limitation of disability require long-term follow-up: special studies are needed to identify the effect of care, which is not immediately apparent. . . .

- The public has high expectations of modern medical care but also has difficulty understanding its complexity: providers must demonstrate accountability to the public [1983, p. 5].

The overall thrust here is that a valid Quality Assurance process is needed to assure the effectiveness and appropriateness of care and to make providers publicly accountable. But what are we specifically trying to accomplish in setting our sights on these broad objectives?

A Working Definition of "Quality"

Any discussion on the aims of a process intended to assure quality must spring from a common understanding of what "quality" really means. Even so, a fundamental problem in ambulatory care today is that few programs have made the effort to actively articulate what they mean by this term. Some have made the conscious decision not to agonize over such a definition, feeling that this process is essentially an academic exercise. However, these organizations may find themselves floundering as they attempt to put together a functional assessment program, since without a basic understanding of the essentials of quality, they will have no real focus for their program development efforts. Organizations that *have* made an effort to define what quality means to them, however, can use that definition to pinpoint the facets of quality they wish to address; these organizations can also argue with more substance about the irreducible minimum below which the costs of their programs cannot be taken without sacrificing real quality.

Certainly there have been many attempted definitions of quality, but most seem to leave out nearly as much as they include. In addition, a number of people feel that quality is an intuitive construct, and that, as with the well-known description of pornography, one will know it when one sees it. One physician has suggested that "quality is. . . like good wine: we know immediately upon tasting it whether it has gone sour" (Munchow, 1986, p. 310).

The dilemma that inevitably arises if quality is perceived as essentially subjective has been well described by Robert M. Pirsig in his book *Zen and the Art of Motorcycle Maintenance* (1974), which is actually more about concepts other than either Zen or motorcycle maintenance. Pirsig writes, "Quality . . . you know what it is, yet you don't know what it is. But that's self-contradictory. . . . But when you try to say what the quality is, apart from the things that have it, it all goes poof! . . . But if you can't say what Quality is, how do you know what it is, or how do you know that it even exists? . . . But for all practical purposes it really does exist. . . . Why else would people pay fortunes for some things and throw others in the trash pile?" (p. 178).

Walter McClure (1987) has formulated a definition of quality in health care that addresses the issue with at least a degree of specificity. He suggests that "quality is three things: *Patient Satisfaction* . . . Does the patient feel cared for? *Effectiveness* . . . Does the health care work? Does it *Innovate?* . . . Does it constantly try to improve patient care and effectiveness for less dough?"

This definition begins to concretely address two of the basic perspectives from which most health care professionals, either formally or simply by the way they practice, tend to try to measure quality; these are the *effectiveness* of diagnosis and treatment, and the innovations for cost-effectiveness (normally called *efficiency*) with which care is ultimately provided. This definition also brings in an element that has taken on increasing significance in recent years — the *satisfaction of the patient* with the care he or she receives.

However, we believe that an even higher level of specificity is needed — and can be provided. In the mid 1970s, the Institute of Medicine (part of the National Academy of Science), in attempting to define a Quality Assurance system, alluded to quality health care as that which is "effective in bettering the health status and satisfaction of a population, within the resources that society and individuals have chosen to spend for that care" (1974, p. 1). This concept will constitute our working definition of quality in health care, specifically in the ambulatory care setting. While several national organizations are now developing newer definitions of quality, and although the definition proposed above was developed some time ago, we feel that this wording accurately describes what we believe to be real quality in health care.

Palmer astutely points out that this conceptual base encompasses five critical factors, which she terms "dimensions" of quality. As she notes (1983, p. 15),

> The dimensions encountered . . . are:
>
> - *Effectiveness.* The power of a particular procedure or treatment to improve health status.
> - *Efficiency.* The delivery of a maximum number of comparable units of health care for a given unit of health resources used.
> - *Accessibility.* The ease with which health care can be reached in the face of financial, organizational, cultural, and emotional barriers.
> - *Acceptability.* The degree to which health care satisfies patients.
> - *Provider Competence.* The core, because it is concerned with the provider's ability to use the best available knowledge and judgment to produce the health and satisfaction of consumers. Provider competence can refer to an individual's technical and interpersonal skills . . . [or] to a health care delivery system and the way in which it functions as a whole.

Here, we believe, is a working baseline from which to address virtually all of the major issues that concern most professionals seeking either to provide care or to structure a system enabling others to provide care. Taken together, the Institute of Medicine definition and the dimensions of quality that flow naturally from it speak directly to the delivery of health care that *works*, that is *cost-effective*, that is delivered by *appropriate providers*, that extends care to *all who need it when they need it*, and that *satisfies* the full set of the customer's requirements. Thus, quality is considered from all relevant viewpoints—from the perspective of providers, patients, and society as a whole; the primary aim of Quality Assurance, then, is to ensure that a health care program continuously fulfills these mandates for quality care. With this in mind, let us examine each of the five dimensions of quality in a bit more detail.

The Five Dimensions of Quality

Effectiveness. While improvements in specific systems and services are certainly contributory, the ultimate goal of ambulatory care organizations must always be to actually improve health status. Therefore, effectiveness relates to the ability of the provider or system to do the right thing in order to achieve the most desirable result for the patient.

This dimension addresses the critical—but difficult and often controversial—area of outcome measurement. While it would be wonderful to be able to say with certainty that a specific treatment always leads to a defined outcome, this is unfortunately not yet possible. There are still, and may always be, alternate modalities with at least reasonable claims to legitimacy; in addition, especially in the ambulatory care setting, many other factors in addition to pure health care will always help determine a patient's health status (as described in Chapter One).

But there is still much fertile ground for Quality Assurance in the area of outcome. Numerous studies have shown marked differences in practice patterns of various providers treating generally the same problems; it would be reasonable to suspect that an equal degree of effectiveness might not result from each. For instance, one study (Johnson, Freeborn, and Mullooly, 1985, pp. 527–528) investigating prescribing rates of thirty-four internists treating the same broad range of health problems uncovered a fourfold difference in the total of prescriptions per office visit.

Much work is currently being done in this area, with the avowed purpose of determining which treatments are generally most effective. This research clearly has quality related implications. A number of national standards already exist regarding acceptable procedure complication percentages, appropriate hospitalization rates, recommended screening/preventive activity schedules, and so forth; these (or equally valid locally generated standards) can serve as the basis for rigorous Quality Assurance efforts designed to ensure optimal effectiveness in the care provided.

This role of Quality Assurance becomes increasingly important in an increasingly cost-conscious environment. For instance, one of today's main concerns in health care quality seems to be the diagnosis related groups (DRG) system adopted in the early 1980s as the major payment mechanism for Medicare hospital claims. The fear is that early hospital discharge and resulting health problems will become routine for our senior citizens. It is just this type of negative outcome that a solid Quality Assurance process can help to uncover through a defined focus on health care effectiveness.

Efficiency. The other side of the equation is, of course, the cost of care. As of this writing, more than 11 percent of the gross national product goes to health care—a sum that causes alarm in many quarters. And the trend is expected to continue. In our home state of Indiana, for example, there is a joint public/ private "blueprint" for the future of health services in the state for the twenty-first century; one of the predictions in this document is that "health care costs will double in the 1990s as they did in the 1980s" (The United Way of Indiana, 1988). Numerous other crystal ball gazers have predicted a similar future.

Clearly, this concern over cost is what has produced much of the dynamic energy in the current health care field. Most of the numerous "alternative delivery systems" are the direct result of competitive attempts to reduce the costs of care. However, reduced costs cannot be allowed to hamstring the quality of care delivered.

At this point "appropriateness" comes into play. Selected diagnostic and treatment procedures must be continually evaluated to ensure both that they have the potential to positively affect the health status of the patient and that the value of these procedures is worth the associated cost and risk. For instance, Donabedian (1985a, p. 34) notes that "physicians who own their own X-ray equipment, performing at least some of the X-ray examinations themselves, are about twice as likely to use such examinations as are physicians who must refer their patients to a radiologist." The implications for both quality and cost are clear.

Thus, another mandate for Quality Assurance is to guide the tough decisions that relate effectiveness to cost, and vice versa; this relationship forms the core of the concept of "efficiency" in the delivery of health care. Day-to-day indicators of system efficiency might include appropriate staffing, timely patient flow, selection of appropriate treatment modalities for privileging activity, and the like.

Accessibility. Americans generally view health care — and, more importantly, *quality* health care — as a "right." Our philosophical and religious heritage virtually demands this view. But do we really practice what we preach?

Many have suggested that we do not. In reality, there is a significant access problem in the United States. Approximately 37 million Americans lack health insurance of any kind; in a system within which health care costs are steadily on the rise, this would seem to virtually guarantee a serious access problem. And this problem can only be exacerbated by the competitive pressures that currently reign in medicine; especially affected are those who simply cannot afford care, or the "medically indigent." According to a Robert Wood Johnson Foundation study (1987, p. 5), "Sixteen percent of survey respondents, or the equivalent of 38.8 million Americans, reported needing health care, but having difficulty obtaining it."

It is self-evident that medicine can assist a given population only if that population can get care when it is needed. In every life cycle, there are certain milestones at which health care intervention is critical; without timely intervention, optimal care and resulting optimal health cannot occur. Thus, it is incumbent on a Quality Assurance system to guarantee the highest possible degree of accessibility. Anything less is simply poor quality care.

Acceptability. The growth in consumerism in this country and the increase in competition among health care providers have caused a concomitant emphasis on what is often termed "patient satisfaction." This is, of course, entirely appropriate from a quality of care perspective, as well as from a marketing standpoint. It is common wisdom that satisfied patients cooperate much better with their doctors; they will also generally return more frequently for follow-up care.

The achievement of satisfaction within a population has to do both with what we term the "art of care" and with various program amenities. The art of care is simply the provider's ability to use the appropriate interpersonal skills to motivate and direct the patient, thereby making care generally more effective. Program amenities cause the patient to want to return for follow-up care, since these amenities result in a perception that the facility is a nice place to be and that the organization's staff are good people with whom to do business.

Therefore, monitoring patient satisfaction in all its guises is a legitimate enterprise for Quality Assurance. This monitoring should encompass, for example, satisfaction with the timeliness of the appointment scheduling system, the on-call availability of providers, and staff interactions with patients; the list is virtually endless. The underlying concept is simply that a satisfied patient is, all else being equal, a patient who is optimally cared for.

This area of quality is addressed with special emphasis by several of our five study sites. One reason is that satisfied patients ensure a better market share. William Loveday, president of Methodist Hospital of Indiana, made a recent statement about satisfaction in the hospital context that applies equally well to the ambulatory care setting: "This is a word-of-mouth business and it's a reputation business" (Walton, 1988, Sec. B, p. 1). In other words, to stay in business, you simply have to satisfy the customer.

Provider Competence. Competence lies at the very heart of quality. As the term is used here, a provider can be either the individual giving care or the organization that enables the provision of care. Therefore, both professional and structural issues are fair game for the Quality Assurance process in monitoring this important dimension. Increasingly in ambulatory care, a major point at which these issues meet is in the structuring and positioning of the medical staff.

Evaluating *provider competence* involves ensuring that education, experience, professional standing, and effectiveness in diagnosis and treatment are appropriate to the care the provider will render. This is, of course, addressed by what is commonly referred to as the credentialing and privileging process. While members of the medical staff can be empowered to perform specific procedures only by the organization's governing body, routine monitoring of the initial and recurring credentialing/privileging process itself should be an integral part of Quality Assurance. (It should also assess the process whereby the health status of individual providers is routinely reviewed.)

Organizational competence encompasses all factors that allow the entity to enable delivery of appropriate health care. This is where assessment regarding clinical/administrative management comes into play; the temptation should be avoided, however, to focus primarily on such indicators simply because they are relatively specific, or because management data are relatively easy to generate.

Organizational competence also involves medical staff's awareness of the need to deliver care that is "whole-person" in the broadest sense. Several years ago, we undertook a study of medication usage within our centers. One result was the finding that patients receiving psychosocial counseling in addition to regular medical treatment used half as many psychotherapeutic drugs as patients who saw only medical providers. There is real evidence that a broad view of health has a substantial impact on the overall quality of care provided.

A final factor must be noted here: "caring." There is little question that caring and quality are inextricably linked concepts. Thus, an ambulatory care staff that actively pursues quality will be a staff that cares; conversely, a staff that cares deeply about its work and its patients is bound to produce at least some characteristics of quality in health care delivery. True caring must be interwoven throughout the entire program; it is the common denominator for all five of our dimensions of quality.

Other Quality Assurance Aims

We have now identified five specific dimensions of quality in the ambulatory care setting; as noted, the overriding aim of Quality Assurance is to continually monitor and evaluate performance relating to these dimensions. But there are also three other common aims in undertaking a formal Quality Assurance effort; these spring from some practical day-to-day considerations necessitated by the changing health care system.

Public Accountability. "Never before, has the integrity of our profession been so challenged by public allegations of substandard care" (Zak, 1987, p. 6). This frightening statement underscores a growing problem in today's medical environment. It is undeniable that we live in a litigious society, and the health care profession has not escaped the consequences; the various malpractice insurance crises of the past decade are eloquent testimony to this fact of modern life.

Thus, an important practical aim of Quality Assurance is to provide a legitimate and documented defense against charges of substandard care. Part of the consumer movement of recent years has been the opening of virtually all corporate actions to public scrutiny; the health care profession, dealing as it does with critical personal issues, is an especially open target. A strong Quality Assurance program can provide powerful insurance against some of the more unpleasant potential results to the provider of an increasingly visible requirement for public accountability.

Several of our five studied programs specifically emphasized the value of Quality Assurance in this regard. Linda Rounds, executive director of the MIT Medical Department, said, "We're under ever greater public scrutiny, both as a university and as a medical provider. Our Quality Assurance program is invaluable in helping us deal with this latter issue." Houser cited, as major evidence for the benefit of Quality Assurance within the Atlanta program, the exceptionally good liability history of the organization.

Marketing. We have mentioned that improved patient satisfaction has the added benefit of increasing market share. In fact, the overall issue of quality in all its forms can be effectively employed as a powerful marketing tool. In a cost-cutting environment with an increasing concern over quality, a formal assessment program that can visibly demonstrate high-quality care will give its parent organization a decided competitive edge.

This is already occurring, and it is likely to gather more steam in the years ahead. For instance, in the field of managed care, Paul Ellwood, the father of the modern HMO movement, believes that "the next phase of competition among managed care organizations will be in the 'quality' arena" (Ward, 1988, p. 33). Other health care futurists believe this will be the case throughout the entire health care field; as one (Coile, 1986, p. 15) has predicted, "[Physicians] will be contractors and vendors in this new marketplace, but price will not be the driving force — it will be *quality.*"

Thus, providers who position themselves now to assure quality to the public will be in an increasingly enviable marketing position as the future unfolds.

External Accreditation. Each of our five studied programs is accredited by the Joint Commission. External accreditation is increasingly being viewed as one way to market a health care program, as well as a means by which to qualify for reimbursement from public and private programs. Therefore, accreditation (from whatever entity) is likely to grow in importance within ambulatory care in the future.

An increasing emphasis on Quality Assurance as a precondition for such accreditation is already under way. For example, the Joint Commission's "Agenda for Change" (1986) makes clear that the backbone of JCAHO-accredited organizations in the future will be a strong Quality Assurance program. Already the Joint Commission has begun the development of explicit inpatient indicators that will be used to make accrediting decisions; it is all but inevitable that this trend will find its way into the ambulatory care setting. Therefore, it makes sense to develop a Quality Assurance program consistent with JCAHO or other external accrediting agency thinking.

Specific Aims/Results of the Five Studied Programs

Southeastern Health Services (*SHS*). The Quality Assurance program in Atlanta has in recent years placed a great deal of emphasis on acceptability of care through its intensive "Service Heralds Success" patient satisfaction program (noted in Resource A). The program is a powerful marketing tool for this proprietary group practice.

This marketing extends both to patients and to prospective employed or contracted providers. A reputation for excellence is, according to Houser, a tremendous recruiting tool and a good mechanism for marketing their referral capabilities; he says, "We have a great reputation with other community doctors, and we'd probably be doing Quality Assurance for this reason alone, even if we didn't have to. And by making quality and Quality Assurance an up-front part of our recruiting process, our true quality level spirals upward continually."

The assessment program has also made significant improvements in clinical care, and that, according to Houser, has helped the program become more successful overall (and, as noted, has provided a good liability history). "The key is, we can *show* our patients quality," he says.

Southeastern Health Services recently sought and received JCAHO accreditation; this was partly prompted by Prudential Insurance, which wanted the organization, as a PruCare affiliate, to be empowered to develop a contract for Medicare reimbursement. This, then, is another specific aim for the Quality Assurance program at SHS.

The MIT Medical Department. This integrated university health care system has a number of explicit objectives for its Quality

Assurance system. According to Bruce Biller, "Because of our Quality Assurance program, the delivery of care is less costly in the long run—and, of course, it promotes real medical excellence." The latter aim is especially important to the staff, both in fulfilling the department's role as a university health system and as a contributor to what is generally perceived to be an unusually high esprit de corps within the organization. In addition, Biller sees Quality Assurance as a significant ally in the organizational fight to minimize legal risk (as Houser also observed).

Rounds sees other values to Quality Assurance from her perspective. "I sit in on the Quality Assurance process to report on administrative monitoring, and this gives me a wonderful opportunity to keep in touch with the clinical aspects of the department," she says. Like Biller, Rounds sees the Quality Assurance process as building staff morale. "The staff perceives Quality Assurance as a very positive process," she states, "and the rotation of staff members through the Quality Assurance committee builds a real investment in the workplace."

The University of Chicago Hospitals. A new top-level emphasis on Quality Assurance within the hospitals system was one result of the external accreditation process in 1986. Thus, continued accreditation is one aim of the Chicago program. The system also places a high value on effectiveness in the delivery of care; this program was one of the strongest of the five in its stated belief in outcome measurement, and (like the MIT program) it has at its foundation a general belief in a "100 percent standard" of care. One of the program's objectives is to make measurable differences in care delivery (and, therefore, in effectiveness). One good example was an improvement of 11 to 17 percent in various indicators related to screening and immunization within the general pediatric clinic, as the result of specific Quality Assurance problem-solving activity.

As an affiliate of a major university, the hospitals system (again, like the MIT Medical Department) strives for excellence for its own sake. One aim of the hospitals' Quality Assurance program is to become an acknowledged leader in the Quality

Assurance field, and to be seen as an expert resource in this area. The Quality Assurance program is also seen as facilitating specific health research activities, again consistent with the functions of a major university.

Efficiency in care delivery and associated administrative systems is also an aim of this program. The hospitals became a corporate entity separate from the University of Chicago in 1986, and was able to move forward financially in 1987. Thus, the cost of care is of major importance to the hospitals system— and, therefore, to the Quality Assurance program.

Acceptability of care is yet another concern. Partly as the result of patient surveys and resulting Quality Assurance problem solving, the clinics were newly recarpeted and repainted, and a program to improve the interpersonal business skills of the front-line staff (telephone courtesy, patient interviewing, and so forth) was implemented.

Washington Outpatient Surgery Center. Cockerline states that "Quality Assurance findings are consistently utilized at our facility to improve patient care, and that's what we're really all about. If we didn't have Quality Assurance, many other things would fall apart." While an original impetus for Quality Assurance development was external accreditation (which was subsequently received), this ambulatory surgery center's overriding concern now is viable Quality Assurance for its own sake. Patient safety is also a major concern in this environment; Cockerline asserts, "If we can't do what we do safely, we've just got no business doing it."

In general, says Cockerline, what makes the program work is the staff's motivation to provide the most effective product. The objective, she says, is a center "where I would feel comfortable if my mother were the patient."

Quality Assurance also has the optimization of staff morale as one of its aims; the sense is that aside from making the center a better place to work, a "family" feel enables more immediate problem solving, and ultimately the provision of better care to patients and their families. "Our staff sees Quality Assurance as one of the best available means to solve their own problems," Cockerline remarks. "It helps them effectively stay in communication with one another, so we don't end up with 'we's' and 'they's' — it's *all* 'we's'. Quality Assurance also helps keep stress levels low, since the more control you have over your environment, the better you feel."

Another concern for Quality Assurance is the acceptability of care. The center has designed a survey instrument to routinely evaluate patient satisfaction with the organization and with the care delivered; this instrument takes the form of a postcard provided to every patient following surgery. A summary of the cards returned (consistently about 44 percent of those given out) serves as one of the specific nursing indicators, and as such it becomes the basis for ongoing monitoring by the Quality Assurance committee.

Community Health Network, Inc. The three HealthNet centers initially developed a formal Quality Assurance process to comply with external accreditation requirements; these centers were actually among the first community health center systems in the nation to become JCAHO accredited. Since that time, Quality Assurance has become fully integrated into the day-to-day operation of the three facilities. For example, audits that in an earlier era produced data for essentially random review now develop data sets designed to feed directly into the highly structured AmbuQual Quality Assurance system.

This allows HealthNet to routinely meet the chief aim of its Quality Assurance program, the provision of the best possible care for its patients. A major goal of our total system is to avoid the "second-class medicine" perception that sometimes attaches itself to organizations that serve primarily the indigent or underserved; it is also, therefore, the major aim of our Quality Assurance program to ensure that our patients receive care as high — or higher — in quality as those who are fully insured or who can pay for private care.

As part of our approach, we address a spectrum of health related needs for the whole person. Another aim of AmbuQual is to ensure that we are appropriately attending not only to somatic needs but also to appropriate psychic and social needs.

Patient satisfaction is also of major importance in our system. We have accordingly developed a system to randomly sample patient perceptions of our system and of care received. Results are constantly fed into routine monitoring and evaluation processes.

Finally, we have structured our Quality Assurance system in such a fashion that staff needs are addressed, as well; as in other sites, we feel that the more our staff invest themselves in the overall system and its results, the better our care will be. It is for this reason that our Quality Assurance committee is fully multidisciplinary, and that we heavily involve all appropriate staff members in protocol development, indicator selection, and generation of organizational standards.

Common Aims and Beliefs. In Chapter Three, we highlighted some of the differences among the five programs studied for this book. As we noted, however, there are as many — or more — points of similarity; nowhere is this more evident than in the aims of these programs, and in the related beliefs about what Quality Assurance can do for the organizations and their patients. These excellent programs share the following common aims or beliefs:

1.   Each believes in the ability of Quality Assurance to actively enhance patient care.
2.   Each believes that Quality Assurance is inherently worthwhile and cost-effective.
3.   Each believes that quality can be both specifically ascertained and ultimately improved.
4.   Each uses Quality Assurance processes/results to ensure public accountability and to minimize liability.
5.   Each sees Quality Assurance as a valuable way to market the health care program.
6.   Each views Quality Assurance as a necessary means toward the desired end of external accreditation.
7.   Each in some way uses Quality Assurance in making decisions on initial and continuing provider privileging.

In the end, all five programs have the same overarching aims for Quality Assurance efforts: organizational excellence and the best possible ambulatory care. Ultimately, it all gets back to "caring," and to the refusal of people who care to give less than their best.

Chapter 5

Structuring a Program and Gaining Organizational Commitment

To the extent that assessment activity helps find real deficiencies and insures their correction, Quality Assurance has the inherent power of a management function.

— Gregory A. Clark,
Director of Adult
Inpatient Psychiatry,
the Cambridge (Mass.)
Hospital

While the process of monitoring and evaluation is at the heart of Quality Assurance, an organizational framework must first enable this activity to occur on a routine basis. In this chapter, we shall address the first task in designing a workable system, the development of organizational commitment for the total effort; this fulfills Step One in our Quality Assurance development model — the assignment of an organizational focal point for assessment activity.

Integrating Quality Considerations into the Corporate Culture

Assigning Quality Assurance Responsibility. The ultimate responsibility for Quality Assurance lies, of course, with the governing body of the organization. This entity must clearly assign the continuing work of carrying out this important program.

Quality Assurance is fundamentally an evaluation of clinical care; thus, it would be appropriate if the person or group assigned the primary responsibility for Quality Assurance were clinically oriented. And since physicians must play a key role in evaluation, it is useful (though not essential) to designate a physician as the visible focal point for Quality Assurance. This, in fact, is the case at the programs in Atlanta, Cambridge, and Fremont; at each of these sites, the Quality Assurance committee is assured of active physician involvement, since the committee has a direct relationship with both the medical director and a physician as chairperson. In Chicago, there are really two defined lines of parallel activity—one clinical, the other operational; the results of these parallel processes are integrated by a joint body known as the Quality Assurance Oversight Committee, comprising both clinical and administrative leadership. In Indianapolis, the current committee chairperson is an administrator; however, the chair rotates every several years, and clinical staff members have previously served in this capacity. (Additionally, the committee reports to the executive director of HealthNet, a physician who is the chief developer of the existing Quality Assurance system.)

No matter what the decision as to the primary Quality Assurance focus, there must be clear assignment of this responsibility (and requisite authority), and all members of the organization must be made aware of this designation.

But this of itself is not enough. If Quality Assurance is to take root, the organization must actively make Quality Assurance thinking an integral part of what has been termed the corporate culture. Quality Assurance is more than just inspecting the organizational "products" and assessing their relative value; it must become an organizational life-style. Anything less will prove counterfeit in the long run. As Guaspari (1985, p. 73) graphically put it, "Trying to *force* Quality improvements into your process through massive inspection is like trying to squeeze the toothpaste back into the tube. You wind up with a bigger mess than you started with!"

Quality Assurance cannot, therefore, be a "tack-on" phenomenon, as we have said previously; it must be integral to daily operations throughout the organization. The entire staff must recognize the ultimate value of monitoring and evaluation and must actively commit to the Quality Assurance philosophy. Without all oars pulling in the same direction, the boat will simply not move forward.

The "Clout Factor." Forward movement cannot happen, of course, in an environment in which the top levels of the organization give only nodding acceptance to the concept of Quality Assurance. The president of the Joint Commission states that for Quality Assurance to be effective in an organization, there must be "explicit top-down commitment to quality and to specific activities to support that commitment" (O'Leary, 1988, p. 2). This is universally accomplished at each of the five programs we visited. While each governing body has explicitly stated its support for the respective program, active day-to-day commitment and support also come from the highest clinical/administrative management levels of each organization. In Atlanta, the president of the corporation (who is also the medical director) oversees the Quality Assurance committee. In Cambridge, the department head (who also serves as medical director) and the executive director of the department actively participate in the Quality Assurance process. In Chicago, there is a specifically designated assistant director of the hospitals for Quality Assurance programs, and the joint Quality Assurance Oversight Committee comprises the highest levels of both administrative and clinical management. In Fremont, the overall Quality Assurance process is managed by the medical director, who is also one of the owners of the corporation. And in Indianapolis, the program is specifically commissioned by the community board, the executive director is the program's primary developer and advocate, and both clinical and administrative management help develop standards and required audit systems.

This top-level support for the Quality Assurance process is what we term the "clout factor." Without it, Quality Assurance will make no real inroads into the organization and will thus not adequately fulfill its mandates.

Allocating Needed Resources

As might be expected, however, this commitment to quality entails more than simply the willingness to make changes within the organization; it also entails the allocation of specific resources to the Quality Assurance process. The two resource uses cited most frequently in our visits were funding for program support (personnel costs, supplies, and so forth) and time. In addition, each organization is actively committed to some type of education or training for those who are to monitor and evaluate — and this consumes both time and money.

Funding. Funding, of course, is the common denominator in all resource allocation. It is by now axiomatic that Quality Assurance is not inexpensive; however, it is also becoming recognized that a *lack* of attention to quality is actually more expensive in the long run. One Quality Assurance writer (Guaspari, 1985, p. 65) has stated, "Quality may not be free, but it's a lot less expensive than the alternatives."

Specifying precisely how much Quality Assurance actually costs, however, can be extremely difficult. The truth is that no one has yet devised a commonly accepted formula for measuring the total of all associated expenses. While it may seem relatively simple to ascertain direct costs for an assessment function with a fixed budget and a dedicated staff, indirect expenses (including the total costs of time spent in quality related activity by non–Quality Assurance staff members) are infinitely trickier. Most problematic of all may be organizational and clinical changes that result from the Quality Assurance process as a whole.

Only one of the five sites we visited (Atlanta) had made any real attempt to quantify the total costs of its Quality Assurance program with specificity. Winer from Chicago, stating her ultimate desire to specify actual costs, said, "It's a great idea — but difficult to calculate at this point." Everyone interviewed, however, stated a strong belief that while the program costs could clearly not be discounted, expense was not a determining factor in the existence or continuing improvement of Quality Assurance.

Thus, it was evident in every case that the organization had made a significant commitment of financial resources to Quality Assurance. While no "standard" cost figures can as yet be generated for Quality Assurance development and maintenance, we have already mentioned that the Joint Commission initially recommends 1 percent of the organization's expenditure budget as a workable minimum financial commitment.

Time. Related to financial expense, yet a separate issue of its own, is an organizational commitment of time. In several of the programs this occasionally posed some real difficulties. Frank Houser, for example, stated that at Southeastern Health Services, "one of our major problems is not getting the physicians to do Quality Assurance, but finding them the *time* for it. And one of our early mistakes was not allowing adequate provider time for the assessment effort." Magda Cockerline echoed this dilemma when she remarked, "One of the disadvantages of Quality Assurance is that it takes so much time. Because of this, we often feel like we may be missing some data along the way."

In all of our study sites, however, there clearly *was* an organizational commitment to providing the time needed for effective Quality Assurance. In each case, there is at least one paid staff member whose main responsibility is to facilitate the Quality Assurance process and to foster its continuing development.

- In Atlanta, the Department of Quality Control, headed by a physician's assistant, assists in ongoing Quality Assurance activity for both the ambulatory and inpatient settings.
- In Cambridge, the MIT Medical Department has a full-time Quality Assurance coordinator (with a background in medical records—a very helpful set of credentials, they find) who reports directly to the executive director and who works closely with the Quality Assurance committee chairperson.
- In Chicago, the Quality Assurance department is responsible for both inpatient and outpatient assessment; this de-

partment, overseen by a full-time manager, devotes the energies of two nurses, two persons trained in medical records, and one secretary to Quality Assurance efforts. Additionally, utilization review, which was recently combined with Quality Assurance, comprises almost five separate full time equivalents (FTEs).

- The program in Fremont, although small, nevertheless includes a registered nurse with the title of Quality Assurance nurse.

- In our own program, there is a full-time Quality Assurance coordinator (also a registered nurse) who divides her time among several ambulatory care units of Methodist Hospital of Indiana (including the HealthNet centers); her job is to facilitate the work of the several Quality Assurance committees, as well as to perform specific program development.

As a Quality Assurance program becomes more entrenched, the time requirement may diminish. A greater proportion of staff time is generally spent in "front-end" program development than in program maintenance. Thus, as Quality Assurance thinking becomes more integrated into the organization, and as the initial baseline data are collected and initial problems are corrected, there begins to develop what Biller calls a "ripple effect"; he has noticed over the last few years that "the need to write action memos has declined, and the call on my time has become less."

But it should be noted that this ripple effect is not likely to be felt within the first year of program development. An effective Quality Assurance system takes time to implement, and an even longer time to effectively graft onto the corporate culture. Thus, an organizational commitment to Quality Assurance must include a long-term horizon if the job is to be done properly.

Education and Training. Education and training really has two components. One is specific training for those actually performing Quality Assurance activities; the other is general Quality Assurance education for all staff members.

Each of our five study sites provides this training. For example, the MIT Medical Department provides substantial one-on-one training for new Quality Assurance committee members, and all new members are provided materials detailing the past year's activities. In addition, each new member is requested to design one new indicator for monitoring and evaluation; this process forces new members to think through the Quality Assurance philosophy, and it serves to help invest them in the assessment process. As another example, each new Quality Assurance committee member at The University of Chicago Hospitals is provided what amounts to a detailed job description, specifically outlining both the overall system and the individual's role within the structure.

Ongoing education for the entire organization staff is the second requirement. In Indianapolis, annual in-service sessions on the basics of Quality Assurance and significant recent program accomplishments are held for all staff members. Likewise, the Atlanta program provides staff in-service education on Quality Assurance findings and results; in addition, company newsletters frequently highlight issues relating to the Quality Assurance program itself and its accomplishments. More immediate and continual education is provided in the smaller setting of the Washington Outpatient Surgery Center; here, Quality Assurance issues are discussed every morning in report, a special communications book including Quality Assurance information is available each day, and monthly combined nursing/ business office staff meetings summarize Quality Assurance findings by specific indicator.

Specifying Roles Through the Quality Assurance Plan

The Plan Itself. A basic element in development of a Quality Assurance system is a formal Quality Assurance plan. This is essentially a charter for the Quality Assurance program, detailing the quality related roles of various organizational components and defining the responsibilities of each. Perry (1981, p. 15) describes such a document this way: "The quality assurance charter is a job description for the quality assurance function. It explains to all affected parties the scope and responsibilities of the quality assurance function. [These] should be stated as explicitly as is done on an individual's job description."

The requirement for a formal plan may at first seem frivolous; however, a solid plan has proved essential in many settings. It is so important that the JCAHO has included the mandate for a formal Quality Assurance plan in its accreditation standards for ambulatory care organizations. Without such a plan, Quality Assurance at best will be more complex and confusing than it needs to be, and at worst will lose effectiveness through ill-defined objectives and overlapping roles.

The plan need be neither lengthy nor complicated. It should spell out the following:

1. *Program Objectives.* The objectives can be stated quite simply; they should normally be those aims formally established by the governing body for the Quality Assurance program.
2. *Program Organization.* Program organization should answer the following questions clearly:
   a. Who or which group is charged with carrying out Quality Assurance activity? (This is Step One in the generic model for Quality Assurance.)
   b. What are the specific functions and composition of the Quality Assurance committee?
   c. How are problems and opportunities for improvement identified?
   d. How are these problems and opportunities addressed, and by whom?
   e. How is problem resolution tracked?
   f. What documentation normally results from the Quality Assurance process, and how is this routinely reported?
3. *Oversight Mechanisms.* These mechanisms address how the organization will oversee the effectiveness of monitoring, evaluation, and problem solving. That is, some person or group should be given the task to ensure that the Quality Assurance program itself is continually effective; this is part

of the rationale behind the need for routine documentation and reporting, as discussed in Chapter Eleven.

Each of our five programs has taken the time to develop a formal Quality Assurance plan, and all find it valuable; several, for instance, use this document as the basis for annual program evaluation. Two good examples of well-conceived plans, one from a fairly complex program (Cambridge) and the other from a relatively simpler program (Atlanta), are displayed in Resource E.

Some plans are of necessity highly detailed; for instance, the Chicago program employs a document that is fully eight pages long. The complexity of the respective plans derives largely from the structures of the parent organizations themselves. Thus, in contrast to the Chicago program's plan, the Quality Assurance system in Fremont is described in a short and rather simple document (a sequential series of policies that are functionally related to one another and center on important Quality Assurance issues, as noted above).

A final note on the plan: in order to adequately perform its function, it must be constantly reappraised and kept current. Be sure that the plan says what you really intend to do; then be as certain that, by actually utilizing the plan, you are doing what you intended.

Defining Roles. Three entities are primarily involved in the ongoing Quality Assurance process: the governing body, the organization's management (both administrative and clinical), and the Quality Assurance committee. Without an initial separation of roles and responsibilities, these entities could at best duplicate each other's efforts and at worst get squarely in each other's way. This can be avoided by clearly defining respective roles; the Quality Assurance plan is the most appropriate vehicle for accomplishing this.

The governing body has fiduciary responsibility for the entire organization, and as such is ultimately responsible for the quality of care delivered. Thus, the governing body has final responsibility for establishing and supporting the Quality Assurance program. The governing body must be active enough in the Quality Assurance process, and must be well informed enough about problem identification and resolution activities, to assure itself that quality care is being provided by the organization.

Therefore, the governing body should actively approve the Quality Assurance plan. In addition, this group should routinely receive reports of ongoing Quality Assurance activity, and discussion of these issues should be noted in the minutes of meetings. Finally, the governing body may occasionally be called upon to step actively into the Quality Assurance process, in order to direct further problem-solving activity, settle organizational disputes regarding Quality Assurance, or suggest resolutions for particularly difficult Quality Assurance issues.

Management also has an obvious part to play in making Quality Assurance effective. In general, management should be given responsibility (and commensurate authority) for four general tasks.

First, it should oversee the program. This means ensuring that the Quality Assurance program is in place and is functioning as intended. Requiring the Quality Assurance committee to perform this activity would be akin, as the saying goes, to putting the fox in charge of the henhouse. And as we remarked previously, placing the Quality Assurance committee organizationally under the medical staff can help ensure that there is active provider involvement in assessing specific clinical activities.

The second task is solving problems. One of the basic principles of Quality Assurance is that the Quality Assurance committee does not actually solve the problems it identifies; rather, this is a function of clinical or administrative management. Included in this role should be the prospective determination of who will resolve problems for specific indicators; such thinking in advance will help depersonalize the subsequent assignment of problems and should thereby reduce the inherent resistance to such assignment.

Third is guaranteeing basic structures and mechanisms. This means making certain that all necessary quality related activities of the ambulatory care organization are in place and are functioning properly, both for necessary data generation and for appropriate problem resolution. Clinical/administrative management—not the Quality Assurance committee—is responsible for the organization's quality control activities, quality improvement activities, and ongoing quality patient care activity (as defined in Chapter Two).

Fourth is helping develop criteria and standards. Management must be empowered to help develop—or at least to validate—the criteria and standards selected by the organization for monitoring and evaluation. Thus, management should participate in decisions regarding levels at which issues are considered real or potential problems, either for resolution or for more detailed evaluation.

Management must also actively support the program. The staff obviously recognizes its control and authority, and its stated support goes hand in hand with that of the governing body in providing the necessary "clout" for Quality Assurance activity. The failure of management to contribute to the "clout factor" can be devastating. A lesson learned in the data processing field is equally valid in health care; as Perry (1981, p. 15) put it, "The failure of data processing management to fully support the quality assurance function has been cited as the number one cause of failure for the . . . function."

What, then, is reserved to the Quality Assurance committee? In sum, this body should be invested by the governing body with five broad powers.

First, performing routine monitoring and evaluation. This ongoing process, as described in Chapter Two, is at the heart of Quality Assurance and is the primary domain of the committee.

Second, calling for information. The committee will need concrete data to effectively monitor and evaluate significant aspects of the program. If such data are not immediately available, the committee must have the power to get them.

Our own HealthNet Quality Assurance committee required the judicious use of this power in the early stages of program development. While a number of needed data sources were already in place when AmbuQual was initiated, some specific indicators required data for which no source had as yet been developed. Therefore, the Quality Assurance committee was empowered to score such indicators at the "zero-compliance" level, causing corrective action. During the second year of AmbuQual implementation, most of these calls for information had received action; thus, required data sources were effectively generated for Quality Assurance needs.

Third, commissioning studies. Frequently the committee, as part of monitoring activity, will notice potential problems; however, sometimes the cause or scope of the problem is unclear, necessitating further evaluation. In such cases, the Quality Assurance committee must have the power to commission special studies.

An excellent example comes from the MIT program. Early in 1988, the patient advocate presented a report to the Quality Assurance committee regarding eighty-seven advocacy cases during the preceding six-month period; it was reported that all cases were resolved without recourse to higher review levels. The chairperson of the committee then exercised the committee's power to commission further study; as stated in the minutes of the meeting, "Dr. Biller suggested that more specific information about patient complaints would be of value in determining whether there were any significant patterns or evidence of suboptimal care. This information could then be transmitted to . . . the Patient Care Assessment Coordinator, for further investigation."

Fourth, directing problem resolution. If, in the judgment of the committee, a significant quality related problem exists, then the committee should refer that problem to the administrative or clinical management of the organization for resolution.

Of course, there may be several official levels before the full Quality Assurance committee gets involved, depending on the size and complexity of the overall organization. Perhaps the best case in point is in the Chicago program, where problems are most often solved through dialogue between a specific ambulatory care clinic and the clinical department to which it reports; problems may also be resolved by combined action of the clinic, its department, and the special ambulatory care Quality Assurance subcommittee of the full Quality Assurance committee. Thus, while reports are routinely made to the full Quality Assurance committee, it is only by exception that this higher-level body is called upon to direct specific problem resolution activity.

At the other end of the spectrum is the Fremont program. Here, it is often a simple matter of the Quality Assurance committee immediately and informally assigning a staff member to solve a given problem. Between these two extremes lies the AmbuQual system in Indianapolis, in which the Quality Assurance committee routinely assigns problem resolution activity through a specific, detailed process and format. The point is that no matter what the variations of specific structure, the Quality Assurance committee must have the final power to direct problem resolution as needed.

Fifth, declaring a problem resolved. This is an important concept, since the simple changing of a policy or writing of a protocol does not of itself necessarily solve an identified problem; only a real change in individual or organizational performance can fully accomplish this. It is, therefore, up to the Quality Assurance committee to determine that performance has actually been improved.

In the program in Atlanta, for example, the Quality Assurance committee gets involved in problem solving primarily by exception, but this involvement includes active review of proposed solutions to identified problems. The committee generally encourages lower levels of the organization to develop and implement their own solutions; then, at its monthly meetings, the committee receives reports of all such actions and, in what Houser calls "consensus and full discussion style," it makes final determinations on the acceptability of these actions.

An additional point should be addressed here about the role of the Quality Assurance committee: the chosen working relationship between the committee and the rest of the organization. Three distinct types of relationships have developed within the five programs we visited. One, adopted by the MIT program, is that in which the committee is almost strictly a process facilitator. Says Biller, "We believe that the Quality Assurance committee should be seen, not as the organization's policeman, but as the organizational consultant for improvements in the delivery of care." The committees in Atlanta, Chicago, and Fremont, while seeing themselves primarily as facilitators, can also fulfill the role of active coparticipants in problem resolution (although usually only on an "as needed" or by-exception basis). Finally, our own HealthNet Quality Assurance committee, while occasionally making nonbinding recommendations for problem resolution, acts primarily in a more distanced capacity, actively enforcing specific standards that have been preestablished by the organization.

In all cases, however, the five committees view themselves as agents of positive change, rather than as "blamers." Biller states, "The Quality Assurance committee may not always be the most popular kid on the block; on the other hand, when it helps to fix things that are wrong in a nondisruptive way, it is usually perceived as something worth having."

Finally, three additional concerns regarding the Quality Assurance committee need to be addressed briefly: the composition of the committee, its organizational status, and the frequency of its meetings.

Composition is important because it reflects the organization's view of how broadly based the Quality Assurance function should be. It makes a great deal of sense to include as many perspectives as possible on a working body charged with overseeing the quality of the whole organization.

All of the programs we studied have at least some multidisciplinary representation on the Quality Assurance committee. At Southeastern Health Services, for instance, the committee is composed of ten professional staff members (in addition to Houser), including a family practice physician, an internist, a pediatrician, an OB/GYN physician, a physician's assistant, the director of nursing, a nurse practitioner, the director of medical records, the health education director, and a midwife. In addition, the committee is staffed by the Quality Control department director, the administrator of the organization, and one hospital-based utilization review nurse.

At MIT, the Quality Assurance organization chart (displayed in Chapter Three) indicates not only the multidisciplinary committee itself but also the various separate reporting committees and reporting services. Through this structure, virtually all professional disciplines within the organization become part of the overall Quality Assurance effort.

Within the HealthNet system, we have taken the added step of actively involving, through membership on the Quality Assurance committee, the supporting staff (both administrative and clinical). Thus, our current committee membership includes (in addition to professionals from the medical staff, nursing, health education, and administration) employees who represent the medical records secretaries, the medical assistants, and patient accounts personnel. This reflects our previously stated belief that Quality Assurance must actively involve the entire organization if we are to get the real benefit of all relevant perspectives.

The organizational status of the committee is also important. If the clout factor is to be effective, the committee must be placed within the overall structure in such a way that its status is clear to the rest of the organization. This is effectively accomplished at all five of our study sites.

At two of the programs, the Quality Assurance committee is a direct committee of the medical staff; these are the two programs operated within major universities (MIT and The University of Chicago), in which professional affiliation is an especially important concept. At two other programs, the Quality Assurance committee reports directly to the board of the organization. Since these are the two proprietary organizations in which the board is composed of owners of the ambulatory care center (Atlanta and Fremont), this structure provides guaranteed clout for the Quality Assurance program. Finally, within our HealthNet structure, the Quality Assurance committee reports to the executive director of the centers, who in turn reports to both the community board and Methodist Hospital of Indiana; clearly, our program also receives its share of clout through this arrangement.

The frequency of meetings should be determined early. Frankly, there is no one "right" answer; the determination will depend upon the active work load of the committee, the size and structure of the overall organization, and perhaps a thousand other factors. Within our five case examples, four of the Quality Assurance committees meet monthly, and one meets quarterly (with active subgroup work going on continually). The key is that meetings should be regular, prospectively set, and frequent enough to get the job done and to keep all involved parties appropriately informed.

Summary

We have attempted in this chapter to provide guidance through which an ambulatory care assessment program can truly integrate itself into the underlying corporate culture—an absolute necessity if Quality Assurance is to establish itself as an ongoing, valid program. Real legitimacy simply cannot occur unless the entire organization "lives" Quality Assurance day to day.

Chapter 6

Deciding What to Monitor and Evaluate

> Management cannot be rational without detailed speci-
> fication of the product.
> — Avedis Donabedian

Now that we have established genuine organizational commitment to Quality Assurance, our next task is to decide exactly
what this process will assess. This actually encompasses three
steps in our model:

> *Step Two*—Defining the overall scope of services;
> *Step Three*—Delineating the important aspects of care that
>   are to be monitored and evaluated; and
> *Step Four*—Specifying indicators of quality that relate to
>   the chosen aspects of care.

An underlying issue here, of course, is *who* should be
involved in decision making regarding these important questions. Here again, there is no "right" answer; the only real mandate is that organizational scope, aspects, and indicators be
specified by a person or group that commands respect, in order
to ensure that the final decisions will be well accepted throughout the organization.

Many organizations find it beneficial to make this process,
like the Quality Assurance committee itself, multidisciplinary;

we agree with this view. For generating real commitment to Quality Assurance, we believe there is no substitute for active involvement in the development of aspects and indicators by persons and groups whose performance will later be assessed through those aspects and indicators. As Biller says, "We believe in developing broad-based investment in the process; we feel that the providers and staff should be allowed to help buy the new ruler by which they will be measured." This is clearly one reason for the requirement at the MIT program that incoming members of the Quality Assurance committee design one new indicator as part of their orientation.

A multidisciplinary approach also fosters total organizational involvement in the ongoing assessment process. According to Biller, "Often programs will exclude either the very bottom or top levels of the organization in program development and assessment. We disagree with this approach. Everyone in the department is encouraged to participate in the process. As an example, one of our custodians recently brought a safety issue to our attention, and then helped solve it. Others in that area got involved through her—now they're all thinking 'quality' routinely."

The Atlanta program also promotes active involvement of the total staff in deciding which program areas should be monitored. Says Houser, "All of our staff was active in the process of developing job indicators for their specific positions, as part of our intensive development of the patient satisfaction program. These job indicators then became part of the code of conduct sent through the organization by the Quality Assurance program, and they form part of the basis for our ongoing assessment in the area of acceptability of service."

Scope of Services

It can be valuable for any organization, either as a whole or through its major component parts, to think through the entire scope of services with which that organization is involved. (This is also a requirement for some forms of external accreditation.) This exercise should consist of a review of the total process involved in the delivery of care to the organization's patients, beginning with the patient's first phone call for service. All providers and systems encountered by patients, and everything that subsequently happens to patients that could affect their health status, should be included as part of this enumeration. Ultimately, this review will define what the organization is all about: who is treated (age/disability groups, disease entities, case mix); what diagnostic and therapeutic modalities are used (medications prescribed, types of surgery performed, behavior interventions, specific medical procedures); what processes of care are involved (assessment, treatment, patient education, counseling); and what enabling mechanisms are utilized (administrative systems, audits, and so forth).

The sum of these items provides the organization with what amounts to an inventory of activities that are good candidates for routine monitoring and evaluation through the Quality Assurance process. This can take many forms, from single, detailed listings to a combination of the organization's mission statement, provider protocols, and so on. The real key here is that the organization has in some fashion clarified what it considers all of its "products." Each of our five programs has in some manner addressed this task; examples of scope of service reviews from several of these programs are included as Resource B.

Structure, Process, and Outcome Assessment

After the scope of clinical and administrative services has been developed, the ambulatory care organization will next need to specify important aspects of care, as well as indicators of quality for each of those aspects. In decisions concerning what an organization should specifically and routinely monitor and evaluate, there are three major approaches from which to choose; each will lead the organization to a different set of aspects and indicators. One approach is to evaluate the *structure* of care delivery; this basically deals with the resources that enable provision of care (see Resource D). Another possible approach is to assess the *process* of the delivery of care; this addresses specific actions involved in care delivery. Finally, it is possible to evaluate *outcome*, the actual results of the care delivered.

Structural Evaluation. All that is needed for structural evaluation is general agreement regarding which specific parts of the structure contribute to quality care, as well as a consensus regarding the organization's standards for these structural pieces. Systems that contribute to the quality of care (continuing education, job descriptions, appropriate policies, and so forth) are all structural components that should be routinely evaluated. As another example, the credentialing system is arguably one of the single most important structural elements of an ambulatory care program, and it should therefore be a top priority for monitoring and evaluation.

A word of caution, however: be careful not to monitor *only* structure. Since this is a relatively simple approach to Quality Assurance, it is an enticing notion to do structural evaluation alone; however, good structure does not necessarily indicate good process or good outcome. Also, it is essential that structural requirements not be unnecessarily rigid, as this severely hampers flexibility in care delivery. In general, it is by now conventional wisdom that while structure is certainly important, it by no means assures quality by itself; that is, it is necessary but not sufficient.

Process Evaluation. Generally, process evaluation presumes a somewhat more direct and defined relationship with the actual outcome of care; it also deals with easily observable clinical activity, with which many providers tend to feel most comfortable. Therefore, process evaluation is a popular approach, especially for provider-driven activities such as peer review. Clinical protocols are essentially written descriptions of acceptable process, and as such they can serve as valuable audit sources for clinical Quality Assurance. Also, many of the national criteria used for assessment by several of our five study programs are process factors (for example, pediatric immunization schedules).

Behind all of this, of course, lies the implicit assumption that if we follow our protocols or hew to national (or self-developed) process standards, then we will be able to achieve desired outcomes for our patients. There is an assumed cause-and-effect relationship between our treatment plans and a positive impact on health status. The fact is, however, that surprisingly few of the standard diagnostic and therapeutic procedures utilized in the ambulatory care setting have been rigorously demonstrated to be specifically related to desired outcomes. Often a direct relationship between a change in health status and our treatment plan is less than clear, less than direct, or perhaps even less than real.

Donabedian (1985a, p. 242) reports on one study involving patients with selected clinical conditions. The study observed levels of conformance with clinical process criteria that had been generated by a group of seven specialists for each diagnostic category. It was found that in only about 2 percent of the cases did the care rendered conform to all applicable criteria. Even more startling is another of the study's findings; as Donabedian notes, "It is sobering indeed to realize that zero conformance is the single most frequently observed value."

There are some other inherent problems with process evaluation in the ambulatory care setting, as well. Norms themselves often change over time. The appropriate process for treating peptic ulcers ten years ago would raise more than a few eyebrows today. Established processes and related standards must therefore be consistent with currently acceptable practice patterns.

Opinions often vary—frequently with justification—on even current norms. Any doubt about this can be quickly dispelled by attempting to get virtually any group of physicians to readily agree on a treatment protocol for diabetes. It is largely for this reason that a team approach to process evaluation can be quite valuable.

In most cases, process assessment focuses on the purely technical aspects of care and omits such critical factors as accessibility or nontechnical "art of caring" issues. These latter issues can be more visible in the ambulatory care setting than in the generally more "high tech" inpatient environment.

Even with these difficulties, however, process evaluation can still be quite valuable. And until we learn more about how to perform truly effective outcome evaluation, this approach (with its presumed relationships to outcome, which are generally more direct than most links of structure to outcome) may be the best we can do.

Finally, we should make special note of a specific type of process evaluation that in a cost-conscious environment is becoming ever more visible: appropriateness of care. It is axiomatic that the process of care should be appropriate to the patient's condition. Implicit here is the assumption that such care is the "right" care, and that the patient is not undertreated. The latter element should be, for example, a primary consideration when assessing process in a managed care environment; in this setting, a major focus must be placed on ensuring that undertreatment does not occur. As one unidentified reviewer of our manuscript noted, Quality Assurance programs must increasingly address errors of clinical omission, as well as errors of commission.

However, an appropriate process will also guard against *overtreatment*, as well. One physician has observed (Bertram, 1985, p. 364), "Unnecessary care exposes patients to risks without offering compensating benefits. It squanders limited health care resources."

Unnecessary care is also expensive to produce, and for that reason it has received significant attention from providers who are actively interested in cost control. Clearly a managed-care institution, as one example, would likely be acutely interested in the appropriateness of care issue as it pertains to expensive practice variations; such an institution would thus be concerned with regular evaluation of this particular process of care, which involves utilization of services. Such is the case, for example, at the Atlanta program, which derives a substantial portion of its revenues from managed care. At this site, a separate subcommittee for specific utilization review activity is an

integral part of the structure of the Quality Assurance committee. Likewise, at the MIT Medical Department (where prepaid
care also provides major revenues), a utilization review committee reports directly to the Quality Assurance committee on
matters of appropriateness in the process of care.

Outcome Evaluation. Every Quality Assurance program should
ultimately strive to evaluate outcomes. Unfortunately, however,
this is often difficult, especially in the ambulatory care setting.
Significantly more research is needed to better tie desired outcomes to specific structures and processes of care.

Some of the difficulties in outcome evaluation remain out
of our control, due in part to the nature of ambulatory care.

- We see many self-limited conditions that will resolve themselves with or without therapy; thus, our intervention may
  not really affect outcome.
- Current treatment for many chronic conditions is only par-
  tially effective; therefore, by definition, outcome is compro-
  mised from the outset.
- The natural history of many chronic conditions is not understood well enough to allow for real evaluation of the
  effectiveness of specific interventions.
- The length of time involved in the history of many ambulatory (especially chronic) conditions makes short-term
  judgments of outcome difficult at best.
- Many of the patients in the ambulatory care setting are
  "worried but well." What is the desired outcome for these
  patients?
- Ambulatory care patients are often difficult to follow routinely; thus, outcome evaluation can sometimes be unduly
  expensive or time consuming.
- There are so many external variables in the lives of most
  ambulatory care patients (including their own volition regarding treatment plans and life-styles) that outcome may
  be only indirectly related to the health care received.

All of these challenges are, however, eminently worth
meeting head-on, since outcome is really quality's "bottom line"

in the health care environment. Outcome is, in fact, significant enough for the head of the Health Care Financing Administration to go on public record (McIlrath, 1988, p. 44) with his belief that $150 million should be made available for the rigorous study of specific outcomes for procedures (in hopes, of course, of eliminating payment for those treatments shown to be relatively less effective).

It is, however, commonly agreed that outcome by itself is not sufficient to enable judgments of overall quality. An inescapable fact of organizational life is that both structural and process based factors will also continue to be significant contributors to total quality levels. Another caveat regarding outcome is that organizational certainty must exist regarding precisely what is being evaluated. Outcome can, in fact, be of several different levels and types. Unfortunately, these distinctions are not now generally made in common dialogue; thus, the parties to any discussion on "outcome assessment" could easily hold different images of what is being referenced.

As stated in an audit systems manual published through HealthNet (Benson and Van Osdol, 1987, p. 82), "When designing an Outcome Audit, it is important to establish the targeted level of the outcome. For instance, a diabetic outcome audit can be done at several levels. A *primary* outcome might be to look at blood sugar levels. A *secondary*, and more significant, outcome might be to look at the complication rate. (What percentage of our patients develop significant vascular complications?) A *tertiary* level might be to look at outcomes in terms of functional longevity." Thus, primary outcomes deal with direct observable results of treatment, secondary outcomes deal with visible complications of treatment, and tertiary outcomes deal with the basic issue of the long-term difference the care made in the patient's life. All are valid for assessment, but the level of outcome being addressed should be specified and well understood.

Donabedian (1987, Figure 5) has suggested four broad categories of outcome appropriate to the health care environment: health status, health related knowledge, health related behavior, and satisfaction with care. All of these types are clearly

relevant to ambulatory care; again, the specific type being addressed must be made clear to all appropriate parties.

Note that we have once again encountered the notion of
patient satisfaction. With the growing emphasis in health care
on "market share," red carpet treatment is becoming the rule,
and the amenities of care are being increasingly stressed. From
an outcome standpoint this is entirely appropriate, since it is
well recognized that a satisfied patient is likely to be more
motivated to follow a treatment plan and to otherwise work with
the doctor to improve health. Patient satisfaction also serves as a
good example of a facet of care that, although generally addressed through administrative systems, nevertheless has a likely
impact on clinical care and outcome.

All of our five surveyed sites put strong emphasis on this
outcome issue of patient satisfaction. As we have noted, the
intensive "Service Heralds Success" program in Atlanta was professionally developed over the course of several years and includes virtually the entire organization. In Fremont, the Washington Outpatient Surgery Center provides a mail-back
postcard to each patient, then tracks both return rates and the
trends shown in the comments made. And at HealthNet, we have
developed a program to randomly sample data on twenty-eight
separate patient satisfaction issues; this "Give Us a Grade" system
uses the "*A–F*" school grading structure familiar to virtually all
of our patients. We routinely assess the summary results of
patient comments and take action as needed; the data then feed
directly into our AmbuQual Quality Assurance system.

However, while patient satisfaction is important, it can
lead to a possible "sidetracking" of other quality issues if it
receives too great an emphasis. Arnold Weinberg, head of the
MIT Medical Department, believes, "We sometimes need to identify what is really driving us—our patients and their specific
expectations, or true quality patient care." Patient satisfaction
issues must be kept in perspective and viewed as only one
avenue toward an overall review of true quality.

Choosing an Approach. There are, then, three viable approaches
to quality review in an ambulatory care organization. But which

to use? Ultimately, the answer depends upon the desired results and the state of evolution of the organization itself. However, it is clear that the answer does *not* lie in the selection of only one approach. Ultimately, all are necessary but insufficient by themselves.

The real key here is linkage among and between the three approaches—that is, a likely cause-and-effect relationship among and between structure, process, and outcome. Donabedian (1987, p. 15) remarks, "[There] is a proven or presumed relationship among these approaches, so that 'good' structure increases the probability of 'good' process. . . . Similarly, if the outcomes are good, one should be able to infer a higher probability that the antecedent process was good." Thus, while the most visible current emphasis is on outcome evaluation, the best Quality Assurance programs will use all three approaches.

Our five study sites all use some combination of approaches for their Quality Assurance activity, even though they employ them to differing degrees.

1. In Atlanta, primarily since this program is in transition to a more formal Quality Assurance system, the main emphasis is on structure and process evaluation.
2. In Cambridge, there is relatively less structural assessment and a moderate amount of process work; however, most of the active emphasis is on outcome.
3. In Chicago, the program is consciously moving toward maximum use of outcome evaluation, in the belief that this is both the best single measure of care and the wave of the future for continuing external accreditation. Even so, the program still spends much energy on process review; for instance, a major objective is 100 percent review of selected procedures, and drug use evaluation receives significant emphasis.
4. In Fremont, the small size and close working relationships lend themselves to immediate process evaluation on a daily basis as well as to high outcome visibility.
5. In Indianapolis, the AmbuQual program actively involves all three approaches. Strong structural assessment is ad-

dressed, in order to make the system as replicable as possible in other settings; in addition, we are moving toward ever-increasing outcome evaluation. As a practical matter, however, the process approach is currently the strongest component (as seems to be the case for the health care field nationally).

Selection of Important Aspects of Care

Following the scope of services review and the selection of approaches to assessment, the next task is to choose those important aspects of care to be routinely monitored and evaluated and, subsequently, to select indicators of quality that flow more or less naturally from these aspects of care. The real key to the relationship between "aspects" and "indicators" is nothing more than the breadth of the respective terms. (Regardless of the specific terminology employed, each of the five programs addresses this idea.) Thus, rather broad components of care (aspects) must be linked with narrower facets of care (indicators) within these broader components; the indicators must somehow be capable of being measured and evaluated for "goodness." One aspect of care may comprise several indicators of quality; any one indicator, however, is essentially a subunit of an aspect and should normally relate only to that single aspect.

As in other areas of Quality Assurance, historical variations in terminology have caused unnecessary confusion with respect to aspects and indicators. Thus, what some until relatively recently called "indicators" are now termed "aspects," and what were often termed "monitors" are now called "indicators." In addition, the word "monitor" itself has been transformed from a noun, as in "a monitor of care," to a verb, as in "to monitor and evaluate." And as we have noted, we have seen organizations that even mix these terms internally, referring virtually interchangeably to aspects, indicators, and monitors while in truth addressing the same issue. This state of flux, although it may be a natural companion to ongoing conceptual development, needlessly complicates the field. We believe that loosely defined terminology cultivates imprecise thinking and that the intellectual discipline required by Quality Assurance demands a common lexicon. Thus, as a starting point, we have included as Resource D a glossary reflecting what seems to be a growing consensus regarding terminology.

A good clarifying step in Quality Assurance development is generation of a written list of selected aspects of care, with specific delineation of all related indicators of quality; this list, if the entire organization understands it well, will do much to demystify Quality Assurance, especially at lower staff levels. This, for instance, is what we have done through our AmbuQual system. As Chapter Nine fully describes, AmbuQual includes a chart of all indicators to be monitored, clearly organized by related aspects. The AmbuQual document also precisely defines standards and data sources for each indicator. The overall system is thereby visibly integrated and made relatively simple to conceptualize; this also makes AmbuQual readily replicable. (Some examples of selected aspects and indicators from our study sites are displayed in Resource C.)

How, then, should these broad aspects of care be selected? While there are a number of viable possibilities, we again suggest convening a representative group of well-respected individuals to make the initial selection. Some commonly recognized "brainstorming" mechanism (such as the nominal group or Delphi processes) can be used to effectively narrow the field of aspect candidates. The participants in this process must then finally decide which of the organization's activities are ultimately the most important to monitor. Generally, these will be activities that occur most frequently, are subject to greatest or most significant error, or have the greatest potential impact on the health status of the organization's patients. Another wording of these ideas is the Joint Commission's notion (as discussed in Chapter Two) that priority for monitoring and evaluation should be given to "high-volume, high-risk, or problem-prone aspects of care."

Administrative/Management Review. As we have noted, while the primary focus of Quality Assurance in any health care enterprise must always remain on clinical patient care, management factors simply cannot help but affect clinical quality—and thus have the potential to impact patient health status. Therefore, such factors must be considered in the selection of important aspects of care (and related indicators of quality). Administrative/managerial activities essentially *enable* care, which most probably could not be provided as systematically, efficiently, or acceptably without them; they can also have a direct impact on the accessibility of care. Thus, the judicious selection of non-clinical services as candidates for ongoing assessment is an essential part of a viable Quality Assurance development process.

This is recognized, for example, by the JCAHO in its "Agenda for Change" (1986, p. 2); the Joint Commission states, "Clinical excellence . . . relies upon and is supported by quality in the organizational environment—the managerial context within which patient care is delivered. Both clinical and organizational excellence are the essential components of quality. . . ." JCAHO goes on to note that by paying more specific attention to measuring both clinical quality and organizational quality, we may develop better information on the relationship of the structures and processes of care to resulting outcomes.

Administrative/management issues are specifically reviewed by each of our five studied programs. Structurally, however, the approaches differ. At one end of the spectrum are the programs in Chicago and Fremont; in both of these systems, as Chapter Three's respective organization charts show, there is a clear organizational split between the functions that oversee assessment of clinical quality and administrative quality.

At The University of Chicago Hospitals, there are within the overall Quality Assurance framework a medical staff quality committee and a clinical operations committee. The link between these groups is the Quality Assurance oversight committee, comprising top-level clinical and administrative managers from the overall organization.

In Fremont, several organizational elements simultaneously evaluate these differing quality issues. The director of nursing and the medical director address clinical issues, while the administrator assesses business office functions and medical records completeness. Each group then reports its findings to the Quality Assurance committee, which acts as needed on behalf of the board.

At various points toward the other end of the spectrum are the remaining programs. (A look back at the organization charts in Chapter Three will help in understanding these structures through which the twin issues of clinical and administrative quality are addressed.) In some fashion, either through a specific subcommittee structure or through the inclusion of both operational and clinical managers in the group performing Quality Assurance functions, the programs in Atlanta, Cambridge, and Indianapolis actively integrate these two elements at the day-to-day working level of the Quality Assurance process.

The selection of significant aspects of care, both clinical and administrative, has been well addressed in a number of ways at our study sites. At The University of Chicago Hospitals, the Quality Assurance program recently received increased top-level emphasis, and specific choices had to be made regarding where to put available energy and resources. Says Winer, "The Quality Assurance office put most of its staff time and its efforts into areas with the greatest possible utilization and where the greatest improvements in care were likely." In so doing, the program at the ambulatory care level chose to concentrate on periodic assessment of selected "high-volume, high-risk" procedures and related complications, as documented on a specific semiannual assessment form (displayed in Chapter Nine).

Special diagnostic categories may be selected; at Health-Net, for example, as a result of monitoring diagnosis/treatment appropriateness for hypertensive patients, we recently performed a special study on these patients (the results of which will be noted later).

Critical events may be selected; the Fremont program has, for example, specified postsurgery hospital admissions as one major area for assessment.

In Cambridge, in addition to numerous clinical aspects, administrative aspects such as continuity of care (defined by such indicators as assignment of personal physicians to HMO patients) are factored into overall quality review.

Regardless of how aspects are selected or the specific aspects that are ultimately chosen, we have one strong suggestion for developing programs: start simple. We suggest not attempting to become "world class" in the first year; select a few of what are clearly the most significant aspects, develop the ability to assess those well, then add to the aspect list over time at the organization's own comfort level (but, of course, with all due speed). This is precisely the approach being used within the program in Atlanta, where the annual work plan, developed to support the transition to a more formalized Quality Assurance system, notes a few basic aspects and indicators for implementation during a one-year period. It also calls for specific suggestions for future development of aspects and indicators, signaling the organization's intent to expand the aspect list at an appropriate yet comfortable pace.

In addition, one specific aspect of care being addressed in Atlanta appears to be growing in significance at a national level; this is the function of risk management, under which Southeastern Health Services lists such indicators as infection control, incident reporting, and so forth. Increasing attention to the risk management process was also noted in Cambridge, Chicago, and Fremont; additionally, the AmbuQual program already includes an explicit set of aspects and indicators directly related to this function.

Let us now look at a specific example of how an aspect of care might be selected. We will presume that one service identified by a hypothetical organization was the prescribing of needed medications. Through the nominal group "brainstorming" process, a representative body of staff members decides that this should be considered a possible "important aspect of care" for ongoing review.

The group subsequently determines that drug prescribing is, in this particular organization, decidedly "high volume." Further, it concludes that the possibility of significant harm from faulty prescribing or inadequate attention to drug interactions or reactions makes this de facto a "high-risk" area. The group then locates a research project that concludes that of patients of selected general practitioners, those receiving two or more prescriptions per visit received at least one prescription for a drug categorized by the Food and Drug Administration (FDA) as "not recommended" (Donabedian, 1985a, pp. 56–57). Thus, this area also meets the test of being potentially "problem-prone." (It should be noted, however, that it is not necessary to meet all three tests to be considered an important aspect of care; often meeting only one is sufficient.)

Through these deliberations, the group decides that the broad area of drug prescribing is indeed highly important and should receive ongoing monitoring and evaluation. Therefore, "medication safety" is formally selected as an organizational aspect of care for Quality Assurance activity.

Selection of Indicators of Quality

As noted, an indicator is simply a measurable component of an aspect, something that can be actively monitored and evaluated in order to ascertain how the organization is doing in selected important areas. An indicator is essentially a subset of an aspect, and it is routinely measured through recourse to criteria and standards that have been actively adopted by the institution. (Sample indicators from our study sites are displayed in Resource C.)

Indicators can serve both as "screens" for more in-depth evaluation and as immediate determinants of clear existing problems; they can also address either aggregated data over time (that is, trends) or significant individual events. The technology for developing and measuring such indicators in nationally standardized fashion is at hand, and future external accreditation decisions will doubtless depend on an organization's development of appropriate specific indicators and on its performance relative to them.

The utility (and ramifications) of nationally recognized indicators is potentially immense. Performance on such indicators could, at the lowest level, provide ongoing information to any ambulatory care organization regarding its strengths and needs. At a higher level, especially if adjusted for local factors whenever appropriate, indicator data could serve to show an organization how it stood relative to the clinical and organizational performance of other similar providers. Finally, of course, such data could be used to set national reimbursement policies.

The selection of appropriate indicators can basically follow the same general process that was described for the selection of aspects; that is, a representative group using recognized brainstorming techniques could deliberate as needed to develop one or more related indicators for each aspect selected previously. Here again, a developing program should endeavor not to bite off more than it can reasonably chew; the "start simple" dictum applies here as well, as does the desirability of adding to the initial indicator listing over time. (The program in Atlanta, in making refinements, again serves as a good example. The group's 1988 work plan included a relatively small number of specific indicators, both clinical and administrative; it also highlighted the organization's intention of building onto this list over an appropriate period of time.)

Let us return briefly to our hypothetical ambulatory care group in the throes of selecting aspects and indicators for initial Quality Assurance program development. Recall that the assigned task force chose "medication safety" as an important aspect of care. This same multidisciplinary group might then consider this aspect further and conclude that "adverse drug reactions to medications prescribed in the office" would be one suitably related indicator of quality (in this case, for outcome). Within the same aspect, the group might also conclude that "quality control procedures" regarding the in-house pharmacy would be another good indicator. (The next task for our hypothetical group, the development of criteria and related standards for these indicators, will be addressed in the following chapter.)

As with aspects, indicators can also deal with structure, process, or outcome. An important example of structural indicators, for instance, is in the area of provider staff credentialing; virtually all of the programs surveyed specifically noted use of

Quality Assurance findings in performing regular credentialing/privileging for the professional staff.

The AmbuQual program, for instance, specifically identifies credentials as an important aspect of care; it then itemizes the related indicators of educational background, training, professional experience, certification, and licensure.

The Fremont program also makes an active credentialing/privileging function part of its ongoing Quality Assurance review. The aspect entitled "qualifications of staff" and related indicators are noted as a specific review responsibility for nursing, and the medical director/Quality Assurance committee chairperson is given the daily quality related task of reviewing all operating physician credentials and privileges.

There are also many examples of the use of process and outcome indicators. The program in Chicago, for example, recently strengthened its policies regarding repeat urine cultures in the general medicine clinic by focusing on the primarily process-oriented indicator of patient compliance with follow-up treatment instructions. The Cambridge program significantly improved its repeat film rate in radiology by identifying repeated patterns noted in the process of taking X rays. In Fremont, Quality Assurance findings led to the inclusion of a routine outcome indicator regarding acceptable estimated blood loss (EBL) levels following surgery in both adults and children.

Once all appropriate indicators have been selected, it is a simple matter to arrange them into a schedule (preferably by "parent" aspects) for ongoing assessment. Thus, for example, the schedule might suggest that in January the aspects of medication safety and lab safety would be reviewed; included would be all relevant indicators, such as related quality control policies, adverse drug reactions or lab accidents, or the appropriate utilization of all relevant procedures by the staff. In February, aspects relating to continuity of care procedures and provider credentialing systems, with all related quality indicators, might be addressed. In this way, the organization can prospectively schedule the entire package of aspects and indicators that have been selected for routine assessment.

As a practical matter, each of our five model programs either actively uses or is developing some form of prospectively set aspect/indicator scheduling system. A monthly schedule is in use in our program in Indianapolis, for example; this allows the entire Quality Assurance program to be reviewed within a specified time frame. In Chicago, as has been mentioned, all ambulatory care clinics are prospectively scheduled to report at least twice per year on selected indicators. In Cambridge, each appropriate committee or service is also prospectively scheduled to make a formal report to the Quality Assurance committee at least twice per year. Another approach has been taken by the Fremont program; there, the full list of all aspects and indicators for the three simultaneous Quality Assurance channels (nursing, medical, and administration) are reported to the Quality Assurance committee every quarter.

Of course, indicators can often change over time. There are really two differing approaches among our five program sites with respect to this issue. One approach, typified by the AmbuQual system, maintains a relatively stable set of aspects and indicators from year to year. The thinking here is that once the organization has taken pains to carefully select and document the most appropriate aspects of care and related indicators, these should probably remain reasonably constant. Underlying this is the view that appropriately selected aspects and indicators will be inherently flexible and generic enough to accommodate all but truly major organizational or clinical changes. This general approach is also taken at the Washington Outpatient Surgery Center.

The other point of view is exemplified by the program at MIT; there, in addition to requesting that each new Quality Assurance committee member develop one new indicator, the Quality Assurance committee also routinely reviews all existing indicators for possible elimination. Says Biller, "We see boredom with the process as one of the main enemies of effective Quality Assurance. For this reason, we are constantly addressing the possibility of moving away from old indicators should they become prehistoric, and we generally anticipate abandoning some indicators at each annual review."

It should be said, however, that neither school of thought is "pure" within our study programs; thus, AmbuQual does, in fact, allow for indicator replacement as appropriate, while some of MIT's indicators remain available for repeated assessment over time. And each of the five programs specifically addresses the relevance of existing indicators in some fashion once each year during its annual program review. Once again, whatever works for the organization in question is entirely acceptable, as long as the result is ongoing effectiveness in routine Quality Assurance monitoring and evaluation.

We have now walked through the basically simple (but often time-consuming) processes involved in the development of specific aspects and indicators that will form the basis for active monitoring and evaluation in the ambulatory care setting. While the selection of aspects and indicators need not be complicated, it is nevertheless vitally important; we must continually remind ourselves that the results of monitoring and evaluation can be only as good as the selection of the specific items to be routinely assessed. Biller's advice is decidedly well taken: "Avoid the petty, and never monitor the obvious."

Chapter 7

Establishing Guideposts
for Comparison

> No evaluation of any kind can be conducted without
> criteria and standards. . . . [These] deserve the most
> careful study because through them the more general
> conceptions of quality are translated to actual tools for
> measurement.
> — Avedis Donabedian

A magazine cover story addressing hospitals could as easily have
been addressing ambulatory care centers when it stated, "Consumers and payers are demanding that hospitals implement an
industrial model of quality management. Hospitals are being
asked to deliver quantifiable and clinically relevant measures of
the quality of services they provide" (Robinson, 1988, p. 38). The
"industrial model of quality management" to which the story
referred is firmly rooted in the quality control tradition, and it
rests squarely on the notion of comparing a result with a predetermined guideline. This model presupposes specified measures of "goodness"; it is for this reason that Step Five in our
Quality Assurance model is the generation of criteria and standards for comparison.

Staff Involvement in Criteria and Standards Selection

As with the development of aspects and indicators, the
first issue regarding criteria and standards is "Who should decide?" Here again, our strong bias is to involve a multidisciplinary team that includes representation from those functions

most directly affected by the resulting evaluation process. Clearly, this group must as a matter of course include strong provider representation, since clinical performance measurement is one of the keys to functional Quality Assurance.

However, many providers clearly have no particular love for this type of undertaking; many have traditionally viewed the Quality Assurance process as a distinct threat to their professional prerogatives. And one physician notes that if performance measurement involves any perception of moral judgment, "a strongly defensive reaction is inevitable. Most physicians not only are highly individualistic but also feel that their personal standards of quality are as high as or higher than those imposed by others" (Munchow, 1986, p. 310).

We believe that the best antidote to distrust is the active involvement of providers, through a team approach whenever possible, in selection of the very criteria and standards by which they will ultimately be measured. While provider resistance is always possible in the initial stages of program development, it need not be either long lasting or fatal, as demonstrated in several of our study sites.

At The University of Chicago Hospitals, says Winer, "there was some noticeable provider resistance in the early stages. Some physicians were particularly reluctant to participate in Quality Assurance, feeling, 'This is a university, and everyone is already looking over everyone else's shoulder.' But through increased involvement, the physicians now see that what we really are presenting to them is a substantial opportunity to improve care. The end result is that our physicians now serve as a tremendous asset to the entire Quality Assurance program."

At the Washington Outpatient Surgery Center, the job of implementing standards for comparison was perhaps less difficult than in many organizations, in part because Quality Assurance development and this relatively small organization itself were begun at roughly the same time, and most of the staff has worked together like "family" since the earliest days. Even so, Cockerline recalls some initial provider resistance to the process, which was largely overcome by actively involving physicians in the selection of criteria and standards. She says, "The physicians are all quite committed to the idea of Quality Assurance now — we solved the initial resistance problems by essentially coopting these providers by asking them to be in on the process itself."

In our own program in Indianapolis, initial reactions to Quality Assurance development included basic apathy and outright hostility. But as the process unfolded, those groups that were to be monitored and evaluated were asked to take an active part in program development. This included a long-term process of protocol generation by all provider staff members; the resulting explicit, consensus based protocols then became the foundation for the peer review audits that constitute one of the main data sources for the AmbuQual program. In addition, we recently have begun to request all managers, both clinical and administrative, to annually review the specific corrective action levels for those indicators that apply to their areas. Thus, our program receives continual input from the persons most directly affected on desired levels of quality for every indicator.

Some Basic Choices

Before tackling the task of actually generating criteria and standards, we should first address several baseline choices that developers of Quality Assurance programs must make. These choices are largely the responsibility of clinical/administrative management.

As with aspects and indicators, criteria and standards can be built around structure, process, or outcome. For each approach, the advantages and pitfalls generally parallel our discussions in Chapter Six. Again, an appropriate mix of approaches is generally a wise choice.

Like indicators, criteria and standards can be developed to address either individual cases or patterns of performance.

- At the Fremont program, every case of hospital admission following outpatient surgery is considered significant. Thus, the criterion/standard set related to this indicator mandates specific investigation and evaluation of all such incidents.

- As an example of a pattern focus, the safety committee at the MIT Medical Department reported on several safety incidents, which the Quality Assurance committee agreed had been handled correctly; according to the minutes of the meeting, "the Safety Committee will continue to review incident reports but agreed not to act on minor incidents unless a pattern is noted."
- In our own program, peer audit results flowing from pre-determined organizational standards are routinely reported over time both by individual provider and in summary fashion for the overall program.

Criteria and standards may be selected to focus on either routine systems and expected events (to ensure that they are as intended) or to focus on abnormal events (to be certain that they are continually being handled appropriately).

- At Southeastern Health Services, one routine process criterion states that all infants must have their head circumferences measured prior to their first birthday; the related standard is that a 95 percent compliance rate for this specified criterion of normal process is acceptable.
- Likewise, in our HealthNet program a number of Ambu-Qual criteria state that routine policies and procedures related to selected indicators of quality must normally be in place, be current, and be functional.
- The Fremont program affords a good example of criteria and standards relating to abnormal events; here, every infection or patient/family incident is considered a variance from the desired standard, and further evaluation or corrective action is automatically taken in all such cases.

Actual Selection of Specific Criteria and Standards

Terminology and Definitions. The first logical task is to define precisely what we mean by the terms "criteria" and "standards." However, as with other Quality Assurance terms, there appears to be a definitional problem. Even though these terms are frequently pressed into service, they are also commonly abused; at worst, they are sometimes employed virtually interchangeably.

And we must again briefly address the relatively new term "thresholds"; because we feel its use can cause confusion when an organization is developing guideposts for performance measurement, we believe that a review of our previous discussion (in Chapter Two) is in order here. As noted, we have consciously chosen to avoid the term "thresholds" in favor of the older and more familiar terms "criteria" and "standards."

A "threshold" (or, more accurately, "threshold for evaluation") ultimately addresses nothing more than is usually implied by the more common term "standard"; that is, it simply represents a specified level at which performance relative to a given indicator is no longer accepted without question. The real key is what the organization then *does* with this information. Performance just below the stated standard/threshold could be judged to require immediate corrective action (which would of necessity involve some built-in additional evaluation of the scope or the cause of the problem). Alternatively, further and more intensive formal evaluation could be initiated, to ascertain whether or not a justifiable variation has occurred — that is, to decide *if* a problem truly exists. This latter choice, which essentially adds one more step to the Quality Assurance process, is the route mandated by the notion of "thresholds."

We should realize, however, that the former approach does not preclude further evaluation when a standard is not immediately met; it just does not *require* it. In fact, it is entirely reasonable to assume that an organization would decide that failure to reach a minimum standard on at least some indicators is a priori cause for corrective action, without further evaluation. For example, one indicator in our AmbuQual system is entitled "patient education regarding medications and therapies"; the criterion for this indicator states, "All patients who start new medications or therapies should receive education specific to these new medications or therapies." The standard ("threshold") has been set by the organization at 80 percent. When this criterion is fulfilled less than 80 percent of the time, our system considers it important to initiate corrective action immediately, and no further evaluation is needed to identify the issue as a deficiency.

We recognize, however, that there are many cases in which absolute and unbreakable standards would limit provider judgment and clinical flexibility. It is here that the concept behind "thresholds for evaluation" is truly useful, since it allows for further and more focused review of the actual reasons for which a standard has not been met. However, this valid function does not necessarily call for a new term.

Before leaving this discussion, we should also say that not all Quality Assurance practitioners buy into what the term "thresholds" implies generically. As our discussion of standards will investigate further, some professionals consider a specified lower limit of any sort to be essentially a mechanism through which to condone ineffective performance. Biller, for example, believes that "thresholds are really nothing more than acceptable levels of malperformance," which he contends should not be allowed. "The 'threshold' for quality is zero deficiencies," Biller maintains, "so I simply won't accept a 2 percent error as 'OK.'"

To return to our discussion regarding criteria and standards, then, how should we finally define these terms? Or, do these words, as they are frequently employed in the real world, actually mean the same thing? No, they assuredly do not; while they are closely related, they have distinct meanings and uses.

Simple yet valid definitions come straight from the dictionary, which states that a criterion is "an established rule or principle" and that a standard is "an approved model . . . *Synonyms*: gauge . . . pattern" (Stein, 1975, pp. 317, 1280).

This same source goes on to note that a criterion, serving as a principle, does not necessarily imply any comparison, while a standard forms the actual basis for evaluation. In sum, we can think of a criterion as an accepted *rule* for doing something, while a standard is a quantitative *marker* of acceptable performance relative to this rule.

As an illustration of this notion, let us recall our theoretical example (from the preceding chapter) of a selected indicator entitled "adverse drug reactions" flowing from the broader aspect of "medication safety." Our hypothetical decision-making group might decide that the rule (criterion) for this indicator should, given the risk involved in improper drug therapy management, be that there are no adverse drug reactions resulting from medications prescribed in the office. However, realizing that this may be nearly impossible to attain in ongoing practice, the clinicians in the group might argue that a 2 percent error rate is reasonable; the rest of the group, feeling that it would be essentially unproductive to set standards that are impractically high, might then agree to this professional suggestion. Thus, the marker for comparison of organizational performance (that is, the standard) would be set at "98 percent of all cases." Failure to reach this standard would then result either in corrective action (such as intensified education and training or a change in procedures), or in mandated secondary evaluation (for problem prevalence, practical impact, and so forth).

Specific Criteria Selection. The selection of specific performance criteria is where some experts feel the real development work is done for Quality Assurance. Philip B. Crosby, in his book *Quality Without Tears* (1984, p. 60), asserts that "the best brains and most useful knowledge will be invested in establishing the requirements in the first place."

This also represents one of the points in the development process at which errors are likely to be most costly. One unidentified author (in Benson, 1989), for example, has developed this unsettling scenario regarding the results of poor process criteria selection: "First, a list of criteria will be accepted as being compatible with good care. Second, a study will demonstrate that there is less than 50 percent compliance with these criteria. Third, attempts will then be made to improve the performance of physicians. Finally, the physicians' behavior will be changed and, as a result of this effort, the cost of medical care will skyrocket, but the health of the American people will remain relatively constant. This, then, will be the outcome of a quality assurance system based on the acceptance of invalid process criteria."

One of the chief requirements of good criteria is that they

must be clinically valid, as affirmed through provider participation in the criteria selection process. Simply put, clinically valid criteria will always make sense to other health professionals, inside and outside the organization. But clinical validity is only one factor in criteria selection. Donabedian (1987, Figure 9) presents other major factors, as follows:

- Importance.
- Recordability.
- Stringency. (Criteria and related standards can be set so high that attainment becomes virtually impossible and enthusiasm for enforcement becomes almost nonexistent.)
- Screening efficiency. (Criteria and standards must accurately separate performance that needs further action from that which is functionally acceptable.)
- Adaptability to case variation.

A final thought from Donabedian (1987, pp. 32–33) addresses the important issue of the need to pay continual attention to the relevance of the specific criteria selected: "[The] relentless progress of medicine dictates that the criteria be constantly reviewed and updated. Like a flower garden, the criteria demand constant attention. But the rewards are also great, [because] those who control the criteria of professional practice, through them control practice itself."

Heather Palmer (1983, p. 77) also has some practical suggestions for development of effective criteria:

- Keep criteria simple
- Limit the number of criteria
- Include only minimal essential items
- Require proved effective items or at least follow conventional wisdom
- Ban dangerous and ineffective items
- Ban excessive and unnecessary items
- Allow best adaptation to provider and patient resources
- Be sure content is up to date

Implicit Versus Explicit Criteria. In reaching a consensus regarding both criteria and related standards, the ambulatory care organization must make a choice as to whether each criterion/ standard set should be implicit or explicit. Purely implicit criteria and standards exist in the minds of "expert" judges; for example, these persons would be presented a group of medical charts and asked to make an essentially subjective judgment regarding the "goodness" of the care provided. Purely explicit criteria and standards are prospectively set and are in many instances defined so thoroughly and objectively that even nonclinical personnel could use them. Perhaps the most recognizable example of this approach is the clinical protocol (see the glossary for our definition of this term), which, if properly developed, provides prospective and commonly accepted criteria for "good" care. Each approach, of course, has attendant advantages and disadvantages.

Implicit criteria (and standards) are more easily adaptable to individual cases, and thus are considered more flexible. However, use of this avenue is generally more costly, since greater time is normally involved—time that, by definition, is of the expensive professional variety. Implicit judgments can also be relatively unreliable by virtue of being potentially inconsistent, since clearly two experts might significantly disagree.

Explicit criteria (and standards), on the other hand, can facilitate more precise and consistent judgments, and they can generally be applied less expensively (often using technically trained support staff). Also, the process of developing explicit criteria can itself be a valuable educational tool for all involved. At HealthNet, for example, we have developed more than eighty specific protocols for the most common ambulatory care diagnoses, and this has indeed proven to be both educational for the providers and beneficial to the quality assessment process.

The major potential disadvantage to the use of explicit criteria (in addition to sometimes presenting some interesting interpersonal dynamics during the development process) is that this approach can lead to at least the perception of a certain inflexibility in care delivery. However, this can be offset by the conscious development of *ranges* of acceptable treatment and performance, or by the specification of alternative procedures, any of which would be considered appropriate but not mandatory.

On balance, we favor the development of explicit criteria (and standards); evaluation against rules and models formulated in advance (and prospectively validated by the whole organization) tends to be perceived as impersonal and therefore less threatening. As a practical matter, however, most ambulatory care organizations, including all of the five programs we are profiling, use some combination of these two approaches.

Our own system employs both implicit and explicit criteria. Three formal audits utilizing these criteria provide much of the data required by AmbuQual; these are the performance audit (a peer review format), the procedure audit (to assess compliance with medical records procedures), and the patient satisfaction audit.

The performance audit bases its findings in part on explicit, protocol-driven criteria (arrayed in the classic "Subjective/Objective/Assessment/Plan," or SOAP, format). However, some latitude for expert judgment (that is, implicit assessment) is allowed the reviewing providers as part of the audit process. For example, one question from the performance audit asks reviewers, "Were all diagnostic procedures necessary?" Clearly this question must be answered in large part through what amounts to a judgment call by the audit committee members.

The procedure audit is a series of explicit "Yes/No" criteria reviewed on a daily basis by the medical records secretaries. For example, one explicit criterion for the indicator entitled "initial history" requires that "the initial history form must be completed, dated, and signed for all new patients." Provider performance is routinely checked by the medical records secretaries, and the resulting "Yes/No" data are summarized and fed into the AmbuQual system for comparison against the preselected organizational standard for this indicator.

The patient satisfaction audit is known as the "Give Us a Grade" program. One of the twenty-eight questions, for instance, relates to the indicator "waiting time." We consider the patients themselves the "experts" regarding this indicator; there-fore, we provide them the means to respond to their own im-plicit criteria in this important area by asking them to "grade" our system on a special card. The organizational standard is 80 percent; thus, if routine summaries of the subjective responses from our patients show that more than 20 percent are dissatis-fied with waiting time, corrective action is assigned.

At Southeastern Health Services in Atlanta, an explicit process criterion for an indicator dealing with radiology read-ings states that all X rays will be overread within two days; such "all-or-nothing" criteria commonly mandate further action for all instances of variance. Explicit national criteria also often form the basis for SHS's evaluations of care; for instance, specific Pap smear intervals from the American College of Obstetrics and Gynecology form the basic protocol for this indicator of care within the program.

SHS reviews against implicit criteria, as well. As part of the outpatient pediatric audit, for example, the reviewer must respond to the indicator of "referrals"; one of the criteria based questions calls for an implicit judgment on the issue, "Could this referral have been prevented?" And in the hospitalization audit, for the indicator relating to preadmission process, two of the criteria state that admissions must be justifiable and should not have been preventable; as part of an implicit process, the re-viewer can subjectively answer these questions either Yes, No, or Needs Discussion.

In the Fremont program, the nursing function routinely addresses eighteen specified indicators. As an example of the center's use of explicit all-or-nothing criteria, the indicator en-titled "employee accidents" has as its stated criterion that no such accidents will occur; the related standard is "zero desired." In the medical area, a peer review chart audit question within the aspect of effectiveness of care relates to the implicit criterion that all pathology reports should be appropriate to actual diag-nosis. (Here again, the standard itself is, implicitly in this in-stance, zero deviations.)

Both explicit and implicit criteria are found in the MIT Medical Department's monitoring process. In reviewing the pharmacy service, for example, the organization has developed an explicit criterion that waiting time longer than fifteen minutes is inappropriate. For an indicator on "denials of referral service requests for prepaid plan members," the Medical Department's consultation committee meets periodically to apply essentially implicit criteria to an assessment (reported back to the Quality Assurance committee) of the effects and appropriateness of these denials.

Selection of Related Standards of Performance. Simply put, unanimity regarding specific standards of care, or even regarding the processes through which standards should be set, often does not exist. As Brook and Hohr (1985, p. 714) have put it, "Let us be clear about the problem: We know little about the effectiveness of many aspects of medical practice, so we have little to go on in establishing quality-of-care standards." And even JCAHO may encounter difficulty attempting to develop national measures of quality; as an official of the Maryland Hospital Association suggests, "The Joint Commission is going to encounter considerable difficulty reaching a consensus on what is going to be measured and then defining a gold standard" (Robinson, 1988, p. 40). Obviously, however, standards *are* being developed and defined; if the situation were otherwise, true monitoring and evaluation could not be taking place. Let us, then, take a look at what is known about standards.

Explicit and Implicit Standards. As with criteria, standards can be either explicit or implicit; that is, they can be either objectively and quantitatively specified, or generated situation-by-situation by experts assigned to the evaluation. Here again, we favor the use of explicit standards whenever possible. A specific, prospectively set, and organizationally validated point at which further action must be undertaken can more precisely and consistently define when a problem is truly a problem. Also, a specific prospective standard can take much of the "sting" out of a Quality Assurance finding; the better part of any perceived threat is removed when the finding does not appear to have been generated as a personal issue. Since the area of standards represents perhaps the most emotionally loaded component in the entire Quality Assurance process, anything that can reduce the perceived threat potentially makes the total process that much more successful.

Nevertheless, implicit standards can still prove useful, and they are very much in evidence among our model programs. These programs display varying blends of implicit and explicit standards.

A good example of an explicit standard comes from the program in Fremont. Here, one of the eighteen indicators routinely reviewed by the nursing function is "statcrit controls" (a quality control function). The standard states that "variance from control tests may not exceed 5 percent." If this lower level of acceptability should be exceeded, the Quality Assurance process routinely mandates follow-up investigation and corrective action. In the medical function, one indicator is entitled "presence of informed consent." The criterion states that written documentation of informed consent must be on the center's medical chart. The standard is 90 percent; thus, when there is less than a 10 percent deficiency rate, performance is considered acceptable.

Implicit standards are also employed here. At the time of quarterly chart auditing by Quality Assurance committee members, "appropriateness of nursing care given" is evaluated. The experts (that is, the highest levels of nursing leadership) use their own experience to make a decision regarding the acceptability of documented performance. Another example from Fremont is especially interesting because it typifies a combination of implicit and explicit standards. Under the general aspect of "patient safety," an indicator has been developed for cases of estimated blood loss (EBL) during surgery. The criterion is that there will be no adult cases with EBL greater than 300 cc, and no pediatric cases involving EBL of greater than 10 percent of the patient's estimated blood volume. The explicit standard is that 100 percent of the cases will be in line with the criterion, and every variance is assigned for further evaluation. At this point, the standard becomes essentially implicit; this secondary evaluation is (as with nursing care appropriateness) performed by the health care experts on the Quality Assurance committee, and these professionals draw on their own education and experience in rendering the final assessment of performance.

In Cambridge, it is well understood throughout the program that most of the standards for the organization are explicitly all-or-nothing—100 percent compliance and 0 percent errors. This reflects Biller's personal philosophy that "in important patient care areas, a 0 percent error rate is perfectly reasonable."

However, implicit standards are also occasionally utilized, as with the indicator of department denials of requests for referral services for HMO members. One purpose of evaluation for this indicator is to assess any potential negative impact on the patient's health. Administration reported recently on such denials over a one-year period; the rate of ultimate approval and re-review was found to be 14 percent ("Quality Assurance Activities of Administration," 1988). In the absence of an explicit standard, the report stated that "no problems [were] identified," and that no action was indicated. Partly on the strength of the reviewers' credentials, this implicitly derived judgment was considered acceptable.

In Chicago, an understood 100 percent (or no errors) standard is also the norm. Two clinic-specific criteria and related standards (selected as part of the twice-per-year block sampling of data from each ambulatory care clinic) underscore this notion:

- (General Pediatrics) *Criterion*: Patients fifteen to twenty-four months of age will be screened for anemia. *Standard*: 100 percent of cases.
- (OB/GYN) *Criterion*: Breast exam will not be left undocumented. *Standard*: 0 percent omissions.

Occasionally, in Chicago, a criterion does contain national or local standards of care that are less than all-or-nothing. In the gastroenterology clinic, one selected criterion states that patients over age fifty should have had proctoscopy or flexible sigmoidoscopy within the past five years; the related standard stipulates that no more than 20 percent of such patients are without such an exam.

This program also employs some implicit standards as well. Winer says, "Standards will frequently start from a subjective *feel* that something is, in fact, a problem." When this occurs, expert judgment often determines when corrective action or further specific evaluation is called for.

In Atlanta, a combination of implicit and explicit standards is also utilized. For clinical issues especially, national and community norms often generate explicit performance standards; some standards (such as the acceptable 5 percent variance in performance of infant head circumference measurement) are generated by provider consensus within the organization itself.

In other cases, subjective peer judgments (that is, implicit standards) are used to evaluate clinical care issues; Houser notes, "In the area of peer review, the clinical field is changing so constantly that we feel it's OK, within the limits imposed by relevant community requirements, to be subjective." For other "systems" indicators (most notably for nonclinical functions), the organization employs what Houser terms "quasi-standards," or implicit levels of acceptable performance based on historical norms and ongoing trend monitoring. Assessment of these indicators by the Quality Assurance committee is based primarily on subjective deliberation, utilizing what Houser calls a consensus-building management style.

In Indianapolis, we refer mainly to prospective and specific (that is, explicit) standards through the AmbuQual system. Performance in many areas is assessed by what we call the "quantitative" mechanism, in which an indicator is scored by simply comparing the explicit standard with a number generated by the related data source (a specific audit, for example). An example of such a quantitative mechanism is found in patient compliance, where one indicator has as its criterion, "Patients keep their follow-up appointments" (Benson and Miller, 1989, p. 196). We have prospectively decided that an explicit 20 percent noncompliance rate is acceptable, for a number of reasons. Thus, we consider that further action is needed only if summary audit data fall below the 80 percent compliance level. The only task for the Quality Assurance committee here is to ensure that the comparison of performance with the explicit standard is appropriately accomplished.

However, within the context of broader organizational standards, the Quality Assurance committee itself undertakes a good deal of subjective evaluation (that is, assessment based on implicit standards) for all indicators categorized as "qualitative." Thus, while the standard may be 90 percent for such a qualitative indicator, the decision as to whether that level has been achieved is based on deliberation by Quality Assurance committee members.

For patient compliance, as an example, one indicator's criterion states, "The organization has a well-defined policy by which patients are afforded the opportunity to participate in decisions involving their health care. This policy is written, current, and complete" (Benson and Miller, 1989, p. 193). Although a standard is specified, the determination as to whether or not this standard has been met, especially as it relates to the notion of the policy's "completeness," is made qualitatively, through subjective consensus development by the Quality Assurance committee. This is a good example of a standard that can be actualized only through an implicit process.

Even though each study program employs some implicit standards, virtually all were actively moving toward at least some significant level of explicit standard setting. It appears that the more highly organized and sophisticated a program becomes, the more it will tend to generate prospective, explicit standards. This is entirely consistent with the direction in which Quality Assurance is moving nationally.

Determining Levels of Standards. The level at which standards are set creates quite possibly the biggest difference in opinion and practice among our study sites. On one side are advocates of the all-or-nothing school of standard setting; on the other are believers in evaluation against something less than perfection. While most of these programs contain something from each approach, one of the major differences in the overall "feel" of each site has to do with the respective program's overarching philosophy of standard levels. Each viewpoint has its own justifications. We will not judge the rightness of either approach; again, if it actively improves quality within a particular program, it cannot be said to be wrong.

Both perspectives essentially flow from the same source — a belief in normative criteria/standard sets. Such sets are built on the belief that organizational performance must be measured against what *should* be the best practice; standards result from a conscious organizational decision regarding the level below which care is not acceptable. The only real difference between the all-or-nothings and the less-than-perfects is where they have caused these levels to be set.

Both authors were in the United States Air Force when that branch of the service was promoting a program known as "zero defects" (often ascribed originally to Philip B. Crosby of the ITT Corporation). This label serves as well as any to describe the philosophy of those health care professionals who believe that the only acceptable standard in medicine must be 100 percent. MIT's Biller, probably the most vocal advocate of this philosophy among the persons we interviewed, calls it the "space shuttle theory" of quality management: "If it doesn't really make a critical difference, why monitor it? And if you *do* monitor it, it must make a critical difference."

Another advocate of this perspective is Cockerline from the Fremont program. Most of the nursing indicators at this program have an all-or-nothing standard level, in which one variance causes immediate investigation or specific corrective action. Cockerline asserts that "some of the things we do may at first seem 'nitpicky'—but then, this is Quality Assurance. If we didn't think it was important to pick nits, we probably wouldn't be here."

In fact, this approach can achieve some very impressive results. In the MIT program, for instance, it caused all cases of repeat films within the radiology department to be specifically investigated and analyzed. The result: while the national average for repeat film rates was 8 percent, at MIT this was brought down to an ongoing rate of *.8 percent.*

A potential problem with this approach is that it may at times become too costly. According to Donabedian (1985b, p. 20), there is a point at which "additional improvements are not worth the added cost. A little more quality is traded off for a lot less cost." This, however, can be debated, in part because the exact relationship between cost and quality has not yet been fully specified, and in part because society has yet to determine how much cost is "too much." And, as Biller believes, it may well be that 100 percent standards are actually *less* costly in the long run.

On the other side of the debate sit programs like our own. In fact, HealthNet's Quality Assurance program has no all-or-nothing standards at present; virtually all are set at 70 percent, 80 percent, or 90 percent. Our approach is that while perfection is a worthy ideal, it is not necessarily optimally productive to actively pursue that ideal. As Walter McClure (1987) suggests, "Don't compare against heaven—just against what the other guys are doing."

We believe that this approach need not imply settling for less than the best, simply that the best takes some time to achieve (and that we may never achieve perfection). The total Ambu-Qual program is so far-reaching that it will inevitably catch deficiencies in some functional areas. But with constant attention to Quality Assurance findings, and with ongoing encouragement for the total program to become demonstrably better each year, we believe we can continually "ratchet up" our level of quality over time.

What we have, then, is essentially an honest disagreement among honorable professionals. Neither view is wrong, and as a practical matter most of the five model programs use some blending of these approaches. In Fremont, for example, a 10 percent variance is considered acceptable in the criterion that all charts must document informed consent; thus, even with what is basically a "zero defects" philosophy, this organization can still live with a 90 percent standard in day-to-day practice.

Normative Versus Empirical Standards. We have noted that normative standards are based on organizational decisions about what "should be." The other major way in which standards are derived is an empirical process, through reference to the actual performance of practicing professionals; this is McClure's "other guy." Donabedian (1987, p. 23) writes, "The acceptable standard could be the actual practice of the same authoritative figures whose opinions would have set the normatively derived standard. Alternatively, the standard could be derived from the practice observed in the professional community as a whole, the level being set at the average, or at some other percentile."

As a practical matter, empirical standard setting frequently involves the application of national standards of acceptable care. This is common within our study sites. The University of Chicago Hospitals, for instance, refer to national standards for bronchoscopy and gastrointestinal procedure complication rates. In our own program, consensus-generated clinical protocols include standards of performance derived from the practices of our own providers.

Empirical processes constitute an acceptable and common method of setting organizational standards. The key in adopting empirical standards, especially if they are external, is to ensure that they are indeed valid for the adopting organization, and that they are fully assimilated as the organization's own.

Summary

The development of criteria of care and standards of performance regarding those criteria is at the very core of ambulatory care Quality Assurance. The mandate for this crucial activity is to enable comparison of actual performance against selected standards. The essence of the matter is continual improvement in quality through ongoing evaluation of actual performance. Ernest Codman, a health care visionary who died in 1940, was one of the earliest and most vocal proponents of these ideas; in 1914, he suggested that because of his then-revolutionary notions, "I am considered eccentric. . . [but] such opinions will not be eccentric a few years hence." Hence, of course, is now.

Chapter 8

Collecting and Analyzing Data

Quality should be measured by results.
> — The Institute of
> Medicine

We have now developed the necessary organizational structure for Quality Assurance, selected important aspects and related indicators, and chosen relevant criteria and standards against which to measure organizational performance. The remainder of Quality Assurance involves accomplishing the actual assessment work (monitoring and evaluation) and resolving any problems or pursuing any opportunities identified through this activity. Step Six in the generic model, then, is collection of appropriate performance data and use of these data to evaluate organizational quality.

Basic Data-Generation Issues

Several fundamental questions should be addressed in deciding upon relevant data sources and ways to employ them in the Quality Assurance process.

Precisely What Data Are to Be Collected? It makes a good deal of sense to use data sets already being developed within the organization. Ultimately, a strong Quality Assurance system will make clear the difference between "collecting data only for Quality Assurance" and "collecting data for their own purposes" (to be subsequently monitored by Quality Assurance). The latter, of course, is the desired approach. And since data development is generally the most significant generator of expense in the Quality Assurance process, using what is already available for other "quality related activities" (described in Chapter Two) makes economical as well as philosophical sense. While some new data will likely need to be developed for Quality Assurance, the organization will be well ahead of the game if it can use what already exists.

In the HealthNet system, for instance, the major audits that feed into AmbuQual were already being accomplished prior to the development of AmbuQual itself. The MIT program likewise relies primarily on data systems that were in place prior to the present Quality Assurance effort. In the remaining programs, relatively greater amounts of new data were required for development of Quality Assurance activity; however, once developed, new data sources generally are easily integrated in the developing system. Thus, in Chicago, Winer is actively developing a criteria file (ultimately to be computerized) of various Quality Assurance data sets and other components as they are developed; these are becoming part of the ongoing system of assessment within the ambulatory care clinics.

Who Will Collect the Data? Since data can be quite costly to generate, the organization must pay close attention to who is assigned to collection activity. Wherever possible, for example, collection and evaluation systems for medical records issues should be assigned to clerical personnel, rather than to more costly professional staff. Such is the case in the Fremont program, where the business office medical records secretarial team is assigned the job of extracting and summarizing specific chart-related data. In programs having the luxury of a full-time Quality Assurance staff, these persons often spend much of their time actually collecting (or directing the collection of) data required by the Quality Assurance process. This is true in Atlanta, Cambridge, and Chicago. Clearly, this approach can also be less expensive than devoting substantial provider time to the collection of needed data.

How Much Data Should Be Collected? Again, expense is a major factor in this decision. Several choices are available.

All case information could be collected and analyzed. As might be expected, this can be prohibitively expensive; largely as a result, none of our studied programs used this method.

Full data could be collected only for the universe of all "critical incidents." All negative occurrences (hospitalizations following outpatient surgery, complications following bronchoscopy, and so forth) would be specifically sent for further evaluation. This method is frequent among our study sites, especially those with primarily a "zero defect" philosophy (most notably Cambridge, Chicago, and Fremont).

Finally, sampling methodologies may be employed to produce data considered representative of the entire set under review. Virtually all of the sites use this technique in some form, since it is both less expensive than full data collection and, if done properly, generally quite valid. Decisions involved in using sampling techniques include the level of persons who will perform the sampling and the actual sample size.

In Chicago, a "block sampling" technique allows a full one-week sample of data to be accumulated twice per year in each ambulatory care clinic; this gives a valid representation of performance relative to selected indicators throughout the year.

In the HealthNet system, we collect ongoing "random sample" data on a daily basis for the performance audit; roughly 1 percent of the active charts receive review through this method, assuring that all providers are representatively assessed.

The program in Fremont gives an excellent example of sampling (as in the nursing "chart review") used in combination with full data collection for critical events (a Q.A. log, based on source documents that capture all negative occurrences — complications, infections, and so forth).

"Relevant" sample size is currently receiving much discussion. While a statistically valid sample in every case would certainly be ideal, this is often not cost-effective; the technology is simply not there yet. As the computerization of ambulatory care continues to increase, the cost of totally valid samples will de-crease. Meanwhile, we can still do effective assessment with smaller samples; we need simply to understand that, given the present state of the art, general and easily observable trends will usually give us the information we really need on how we are doing in a specific area and whether or not a problem in this area is likely.

What Will Be the Frequency of Data Collection? The answer here depends largely upon decisions regarding sample size and fre-quency of monitoring. In making sample size decisions, ques-tions about the frequency of data collection will be addressed as a matter of course. Some organizations may choose, for exam-ple, to collect a small amount of data on a daily basis (as we do within HealthNet), while others (such as the Chicago program) may use a "block sampling" technique. How often a particular indicator is to be evaluated will also clearly have a direct bearing on the frequency of data collection; for example, monthly eval-uation would naturally call for more frequent data generation than would an annual cycle.

However these questions are answered, the resulting data will ultimately need to be arranged for easiest, quickest, and most effective review by the Quality Assurance committee. Biller makes this point when he suggests that a Quality Assurance program should "display data so that even a *stranger* could use it."

Specific Data Sources

The Basic Choices. Where, then, can needed data be found? The possible sources are many and varied; an initial listing would include the following:

- The medical record
- Drug profiles/medication records
- Patient satisfaction surveys
- Incident reports
- Direct observation by providers, support staff, patients, other visitors, and so forth

- Claims data (especially as noted in the ambulatory care encounter form)
- Findings of the utilization review function
- Patient interviews
- Log books (such as those used for referrals)
- Appointment books
- Lab reports
- Radiology reports
- Minutes of relevant meetings

Notice that the medical record is the first source on the list; in fact, the chart is an essential tool in the collection of direct patient care data (as well as being required by regulation, for external accreditation, and so forth). For this reason, charts must be legible to all appropriate staff members, and they must be consistently used to document all important events in care delivery.

There is, however, a major word of caution regarding the use of data from the medical record. For many reasons, ranging from the general lack of documentation for interpersonal factors of care, to the frequent inability of the record to verify provider decision-making processes, the medical chart cannot always be considered an absolute or pure source for required data. Donabedian (1987, p. 35) notes, "[There] is no doubt that medical records are the Achilles' heel of quality monitoring." However, this need not be the case; when completeness, timeliness, legibility, and accuracy of the chart are enforced, the medical record is one of the best data sources available for Quality Assurance.

Overall, each of the programs we visited uses a variety of sources for the data required by their respective Quality Assurance systems. At the Washington Outpatient Surgery Center, the policy on nursing service Quality Assurance lists the following specific data sources: "Chart review . . . ; patient satisfaction survey; observations; notification and statements of concern; performance appraisal; medical and nursing staff suggestions; Q.A. log; lab reports; and other relevant methods." The medical record is the primary data source for assessment within the medical function, both for the daily review performed by the medical director and for the quarterly random-sample peer review audit carried out by the Quality Assurance committee. And, of course, the chart is also the main data source for the procedural records review performed routinely in the business office area.

Several programs employ processes for getting specific quality related input from any individuals (staff, patients, and family) who note a concern with the organization's operations. At HealthNet, we utilize a special form on which patients may make comments regarding specific incidents or the perceived need for program or facility improvements; this is considered a valid data source for Quality Assurance.

In Fremont, as noted above, a "notification/statement of concern" program allows staff members and physicians to anonymously file concerns regarding "an event or circumstance which: (a) adversely affects the care of any individual patient, (b) may adversely affect the care of any individual patient, [or] (c) causes something to happen to a patient, family member or visitor to the Center and has an undesirable or untoward effect on that person." The forms and resulting data produced by this system feed directly into the overall Quality Assurance system used at the Washington Outpatient Surgery Center.

Another important data source used in all five programs is the special study. This mechanism enables the organization to focus on one particular issue by developing intensive data and performing specific evaluation on that issue.

HealthNet, for example, utilizes three types of special studies: a problem focused study, to investigate the scope or cause of an identified special problem; an outcome audit, to see what effect treatment is having in a specific clinical area; and a medication audit, to test basic effectiveness of medication by patient, by specific medication, or by disease category.

During one period at the Fremont program, there were three special studies being performed simultaneously: one on the occurrence of nausea and vomiting resulting from surgery; one related to postsurgical infection rates, and one on the uses of narcotics at the center.

At Southeastern Health Services, a special study performed prior to our visit addressed the specific issue of the quality of referral communication.

Routine audits are another basic source of data; we found some form of formal audit activity in use at each of our five model programs. We should note at this point that the term "audit" as used here simply connotes a system for generation of data and does not imply the specific format required earlier by JCAHO for Quality Assurance. Common nonclinical audits include those for patient satisfaction results and procedural charting issues. For clinical issues, peer review audits provide the data needed for evaluation. Because the peer review audit is so integral to Quality Assurance programs everywhere, we need to look at this important tool in depth.

Professional Peer Review. Some form of professional peer review mechanism is used by virtually all functional assessment programs to generate clinical performance data from the provider's viewpoint. As we define the term, peer review is the process by which the performance of an individual practitioner is evaluated against a reasonable expectation of care based on either explicit or implicit criteria. This review is carried out by another practitioner of the same discipline (and often, though not always, of the same specialty); that is, physicians review physicians, nurses review nurses, dentists review dentists, and so forth.

However the concept is defined, we strongly suggest that peer review be actively used to highlight and validate *excellence* in care delivery as well as potential clinical problems. This will do much to facilitate provider acceptance of the peer review process.

All of our five study sites employ peer review audits in some fashion. At HealthNet, for example, our performance audit is a separate system that feeds continuously into Ambu-Qual. All providers (in all primary care specialties) participate in the review process, rotating through the audit committee on a quarterly basis. Randomly selected charts are pulled and reviewed against preestablished guidelines; positive dialogue is held with any provider producing a questionable case, and the final results of the total process are summarized for inclusion by the Quality Assurance Committee in overall organizational evaluation.

In the larger and more complex programs (Atlanta, Cambridge, and Chicago), the actual work of peer review is basically decentralized; that is, each department or other clinical division performs its own peer review independent of other groups, then reports the results to the Quality Assurance committee. Thus, for example, each specific department in the Atlanta program performs a separate peer review, with the goal of at least quarterly clinical assessment by each department; contracted physicians undergo this review once a year.

In the smaller Fremont program (and in the relatively small Indianapolis program as well) the peer review process is more centralized. At the Washington Outpatient Surgery Center, the Quality Assurance committee (six persons, five of whom are physicians) performs quarterly peer review on a random sample of at least fifty charts. In addition, all charts involving certain critical incidents (estimated blood loss, or EBL, above limits, for example) are also reviewed. As a final Quality Assurance check, the medical director personally reviews all charts prior to and immediately following surgery.

It is appropriate here to touch briefly on the concept of "protocols." A protocol is the foundation for an explicit peer review process; it defines reasonable expectations of care against which performance will be evaluated. Protocols frequently (though not always) include diagnostic and treatment criteria, in addition to documentation expectations. The criteria stated in the protocol should be predetermined and clinically valid (that is, they should make clinical sense to external providers).

Although protocols can be highly valuable in assessing clinical care, many providers feel they smack of what is pejoratively termed "cookbook medicine." It has been suggested, however, that when one goes to a good restaurant, one most probably hopes that a specific recipe is being consulted for the entree; cookbooks can, indeed, be decidedly useful.

At HealthNet, we have found protocols to be quite helpful

in facilitating provider performance, as well as in assessing that performance over time. We believe that the following suggestions can do much to help protocols become viewed as valid, acceptable instruments in the provision and evaluation of quality ambulatory care:

1. Explicit criteria should be used, since these are generally more effective than implicit criteria in the performance of audits. Explicit criteria can also help counter the professional fear that often accompanies an implicit process; minimal acceptable criteria or stated practice "ranges" that allow for justifiable variances from elements of the protocol can be quite helpful here.
2. Protocols should be kept as simple as possible. They should focus only on the critical elements of care.
3. The professional staff should be actively involved in the development of the protocols; these instruments will then represent an acceptable group consensus regarding quality care.
4. Protocols unify the diagnostic and therapeutic approaches of the group, and this should be actively used to foster real continuity of care among all group members. (Of course, justifiable variances from established protocols are permissible and should be documented as they occur.)

But protocols, no matter how helpful for some, may never be for everyone. Besides frequently being perceived as the cookie cutter approach, protocols are also sometimes criticized for focusing too heavily on the process of care rather than on outcomes. Biller states, for example, "We don't actively use protocols in the Quality Assurance process—just indicators and monitoring activity." The underlying belief, of course, is that focusing on actual results produces greater benefits than spending great amounts of time on process. This belief can, however, be accommodated by a protocol development process that is appropriately sensitive to an outcome orientation.

Overall, peer review (through protocols) provides a major data source for Quality Assurance monitoring and evaluation.

In order to be most effective and efficient, such audits should be timely, largely random, not significantly time consuming (especially with respect to physician time), relatively inexpensive, and participative; in addition, their feedback to individual providers should be as concurrent as possible. Finally, of course, feedback from the audit must be used to actively and permanently change suboptimal provider performance.

Identification of Patterns

Before turning our attention to ways in which performance throughout the entire organization can be changed for the better, we need to touch on one last issue related to the finding of problems through the analysis of appropriate data. This is the issue of patterns of performance (sometimes called trends), as opposed to single notable occurrences. Both are certainly valid candidates for problem resolution; however, the Quality Assurance program will probably get the most mileage from a search for continuing patterns of variance.

For best overall effect, trends addressed by a Quality Assurance program should be of two types: patterns of real or potential *deficiencies* (which should immediately set off either corrective action or follow-up evaluation), and patterns of *excellence* (which should be publicly recognized and actively promoted as organizational models). It is our strong belief that the Quality Assurance process should be a positive motivator of change, and the value of public praise for excellence is hard to dispute.

The use of data to identify patterns can be one of the primary tools available to Quality Assurance. McClure (1987) graphically made this point in a presentation when he said, "One of the great myths of modern medicine is that you can look at a few charts and determine whether quality is present *in an episode.* . . . This is archaic quality control. Modern quality control is statistical. . . . If we judged baseball players like we judge medicine, a panel of hitters would stand behind the plate . . . watch a few hitters take a swing, and decide whether the hitter had 'quality' or not! Now, I'd hate to have you picking ball players for me if that's the way you did it. . . ."

The message is clear: while individual events will always be important (and, if variant, should not be overlooked), the "biggest bang for the buck" in problem solving is obtained by looking for overall patterns of real or potential problems. This idea is addressed by the Quality Assurance mechanisms in place within our model programs.

At The University of Chicago Hospitals (where computerization is being implemented, in part to locate patterns and to categorize identified problems), several suboptimal patterns have been corrected. Results of patient satisfaction studies in the ambulatory care clinics, for example, focused attention on the need for significant enhancements to decor. Also, according to Winer, a recurring lack of full documentation in some functional areas—a not uncommon problem in many settings—was confirmed; Winer notes, "Quality Assurance provided a good lever to help solve this issue."

Patient satisfaction patterns are also addressed in our Indianapolis program, but we have been fortunate to uncover an ongoing trend of routinely high marks from our patients. However, we have found other patient related patterns that have concerned us from a quality perspective, such as routinely low marks regarding patient compliance. And the value of both problem pattern identification and special studies was recently underscored through one of our early special outcome audits; this review indicated that for patients who had hypertension as a continuing diagnosis, fully 41 percent of the most recent blood pressure readings fell outside of our standards for hypertension control.

The MIT program provides us with yet another example of what can be accomplished by focusing on patterns identified through the Quality Assurance process. As noted previously, ongoing assessments in radiology showed a continuing pattern of repeat film rates below organizational standards. Further investigation showed that the rates could be reduced through certain techniques in working with pediatric patients. The result: the repeat film rate was reduced to, and remains at, less than 1 percent. The department is justifiably proud of this result, and this has worked to give even more credibility to the Quality Assurance program.

The generation of ongoing data and the use of those data to evaluate the organization's performance are the point at which the building of a Quality Assurance program is translated into the actual implementation of that program. This propels us logically toward the next step: problem resolution, which is really "where the rubber meets the road" in the total Quality Assurance process.

Chapter 9

Selecting an Instrument for Evaluating the Quality of Care

> You must suggest instruments that will detect it [quality], or live with the explanation that instruments don't detect it because your whole Quality concept, to put it politely, is a large pile of nonsense.
> — Robert M. Pirsig, *Zen and the Art of Motorcycle Maintenance*

We are now two-thirds of the way through the steps in our generic approach to Quality Assurance development; we have come to the stage at which monitoring and evaluation is being routinely performed and the actual work of solving problems or pursuing opportunities to improve is about to be undertaken. This is the appropriate point at which to make a minor detour from our generic model, in order to address the issue of selecting an overall format, or "instrument," for ongoing assessment and problem resolution.

Such instruments can, of course, come in many different varieties, from highly formal to significantly less formal. While our own AmbuQual system is highly structured, for instance, a developer of another of the five studied programs jokingly referred to the "instruments" in use within that system as "a pen and a telephone." (In like fashion, another interviewee said that her idea of "business machines" included a phone and a stapler.) Memos, ongoing meetings, and phone contacts can, in fact, serve as valid primary instruments of Quality Assurance and resulting organizational change, as is the case in several of the programs we visited. The keys to making these informal types of instruments work are active follow-up, at least some formal documentation, and effective integration into the overall organization and its other systems.

Each of the five programs, however, also has at least some formal instruments in place for carrying out Quality Assurance (generally for discrete functions that form portions of the total assessment effort). Each of the programs, for instance, has a documented Quality Assurance plan (an essential program element, as Chapter Five described in more detail), which basically serves as a formal instrument for structuring the overall program and enabling all subsequent Quality Assurance activity. Other formal instruments are also in use at the five sites to facilitate the various components of the Quality Assurance process.

In Fremont, for instance, the indicators of quality, together with their various criteria and related organizational standards, are formally documented to facilitate review of the total program at each quarterly Quality Assurance meeting. For each indicator, an ongoing Quality Assurance log (backed up by separate data collection sheets) has been developed to constantly document and track the results of Quality Assurance activity on these indicators. Specific forms (displayed in Chapter Eleven) have also been developed for monitoring and evaluation; companion forms document each case of an identified problem.

The University of Chicago Hospitals program has a specific instrument for facilitating the semiannual block sample review of the activity of each ambulatory care clinic. This form, displayed as Exhibit 2, makes the total one-week review of selected indicators a relatively simple and structured task, and it documents the results of this assessment for use throughout the total Quality Assurance structure. A narrative addressing important issues is also required as part of each clinic's semiannual review. Recently, the program has begun implementation of an even more formalized "instrument"—a sophisticated

Exhibit 2. University of Chicago Hospitals Block Sample Report Form.

QUALITY OF CARE/SERVICE REPORT

(Month of) _____

(Name of Clinic) _____

Indicators	Monday	Tuesday	Wednesday	Thursday	Friday	Total
1. Total number of visits						
2. Number of new patients						
3. Number of *new* appointments missed						
4. Number of *return* appointments missed						
5. Number of missing charts						
6. Total number of procedures*: (enter respective complications in item 7)						
A. _____						
B. _____						
C. _____						
7. Number of (respective) complications						
A. _____						
B. _____						
C. _____						
8. Number of patients who refused treatment, or left before being seen						
9. Number of unplanned direct admissions to the hospital from the clinic						
Two clinic specific criteria:						
10. _____						
11. _____						

* Procedures selected should be of those most frequently performed or with an increased risk of complication.

computerized system for storing, tracking, and retrieving Quality Assurance data and results.

Virtually any type of mechanism for facilitating either a discrete assessment component or the flow of the entire program is an appropriate instrument serving the total effort. Here again, the key is that such an instrument is successful within its own organizational context in actively promoting effective monitoring, evaluation, and problem resolution.

The Ambuqual System

Program Overview. In the remainder of this chapter, we will take a closer look at one specific, fully integrated instrument for accomplishing Quality Assurance, the AmbuQual system, developed for use by HealthNet in Indianapolis. While AmbuQual is certainly not the only possible mechanism for facilitating the Quality Assurance process in ambulatory care centers, we have chosen to focus on this program for three cogent reasons.

1. Having developed this program, we are, of course, most intimately familiar with this particular system and the developmental issues involved.
2. AmbuQual is the most highly structured, systematic, and fully coordinated of the instruments in use among the five sites, and it represents perhaps the most consciously integrated approach to monitoring, evaluation, and problem solving.
3. Finally, it is the only ambulatory care Quality Assurance system of which we are aware that actively *quantifies* quality, resulting in numerical indices for both the organizational (summary) level of quality and the quality levels of each program component.

AmbuQual is based on a document of more than 200 pages that serves as a virtual "road map" to overall quality assessment. Thus, one of its strongest features is that it details a highly specific role and resulting explicit tasks for the Quality Assurance committee. The document is laid out on what we believe is a visibly logical framework that makes perfectly clear which indicators fit with which specific aspects of care; what explicit criteria and standards have been developed for these indicators; which data sources provide the input for each indicator; and who is responsible for accomplishing needed corrective actions within each functional area.

The basic AmbuQual concept and the resulting initial document were actually the product of one extremely intense — and thoroughly exhausting — weekend. This frantic burst of creative energy is, however, somewhat misleading, for the fundamental ideas and basic system components had actually been undergoing general development for several years.

Following creation of the initial document, several more years were spent refining the system and its components, performing research on the validity and replicability of the program, and field testing the system in other ambulatory care sites around the country. The result is a total program that can tell us (and virtually any other ambulatory care provider) what to monitor and evaluate; how the evaluation process should occur; who should perform the monitoring and related follow-up activities; what should happen if problem solving is not actually accomplished or does not ultimately resolve the problem; and, finally, what the organization's ongoing level of quality is and what has caused it to improve or decline over time.

AmbuQual has, we feel, a number of significant programmatic benefits. The system is flexible and generic; that is, it can work in all types and sizes of ambulatory care organizations.

It is fully compatible with Joint Commission (and other) accreditation standards and has been highly praised in several accreditation surveys. It addresses all of the basic components of the JCAHO Quality Assurance model (and of the proven approach outlined in Chapter Two of this book). Thus, AmbuQual specifies a job description for the Quality Assurance committee; builds in organizational "clout" for the Quality Assurance program; actively develops specific aspects of care, as well as related indicators and explicit criteria and standards for those indicators; specifies a format for corrective action assignment, tracking, and follow-up; and integrates Quality Assurance information into the overall organization.

The program provides numerical assessments of quality using a sophisticated scoring and tracking system. In addition, it can function either as a manual or a computerized system. While AmbuQual was intended to be computer supported (using IBM-PC or compatible equipment), it can also be fully utilized in the manual mode.

AmbuQual also fulfills the major theoretical requirements for an effective approach to assessment (Donabedian, 1987, Figure 5). Its measures are "causally valid"; that is, most of the structural aspects are generally considered to be actively related to accepted processes of care, and the stated processes seem to relate well to outcomes of care (and vice versa). AmbuQual is, by definition, "relevant" to objectives of care, since many of the indicators are self-selected by the using organization in light of its own specific objectives and scope of services (as discussed in Chapter Six). The program is "sensitive," in that it can actively detect existing quality problems; in addition, by identifying precisely where in the organization deficiencies occur, AmbuQual is both "specific" and valuable in actually managing quality (both in specified areas and throughout the organization). The program is "inclusive," in that it specifically addresses what we believe to be all relevant components of care (including the contributions of providers involved in "whole person" care and of the patients themselves). And AmbuQual is "cost-effective," since it fosters efficiency in Quality Assurance and relies on data that are readily available within most ambulatory care organizations.

The major potential disadvantage of the system is in the area of "timeliness." AmbuQual is, as noted, highly formatted and structured, and it operates on a schedule that provides for active Quality Assurance committee review of each indicator approximately once per year; therefore, it may on occasion not be as immediately responsive to identified problems as more informal systems or those whose primary focus is immediacy in problem solving. However, this drawback is more potential than real in most cases. AmbuQual contains many structure and process indicators, which are in practice the most readily observable and the most likely to lend themselves to immediate solutions. In addition, three continuing audits collect many of the data utilized by AmbuQual, and these audits have their own built-in mechanisms for quick deficiency identification and problem solving. And finally, the Quality Assurance committee actively prioritizes problems and can, if desired, set virtually immediate target dates for problem solving; thus, the committee can enforce prompt action whenever it is truly required.

Parameters of Care. The conceptual framework of AmbuQual centers around ten broad vantage points from which the total delivery of care in the ambulatory setting can be viewed. We call these vantage points "parameters." (This specific term, and all subsequent references to AmbuQual, are found in *AmbuQual: An Ambulatory Quality Assurance and Quality Management System*, published in 1989 by Community Health Network, Inc., and Methodist Hospital of Indiana, Inc.) These parameters were initially constructed through a review of HealthNet's overall scope of services. And we must here acknowledge the work of Elizabeth Flanagan, former director of the Joint Commission's program for ambulatory care accreditation; she first proposed the concept of broad parameters to us as we were attempting to deal with categorization of existing quality related data sources.

Just as the leads of an electrocardiograph view the heart from twelve different perspectives, so do our selected parameters view an overall ambulatory care program from ten different vantage points. Each of these separate perspectives plays an important role in the total delivery of care within an ambulatory care organization. These parameters flow easily from the functional definition of quality (and the five related dimensions of quality) that we proposed earlier in this book.

Provider staff is at the very heart of any ambulatory care program. It relates to the provider's ability to use the best available knowledge, skill, and judgment to produce a desired health outcome. It relates both to technical skills and to the provider's interpersonal skill—that is, both the "art" and "science" of ambulatory care. Specifically included is the issue of provider

competence, which involves such considerations as credentialing, privileging, continuing education, validation of current
competency levels, and actual clinical performance.

Support staff performance recognizes that the daily jobs of
the rest of the staff also have a significant impact on the quality
of care. Thus, the thoroughness, efficiency, and accuracy of the
support staff's work become important issues, along with such
intangibles as positive relationships with the patients and cooperative health care team interaction. In addition to the actual
clinical performance of the support staff, background qualifications such as education, training, experience, and certification
are important considerations, as are current competence, appropriateness of related job descriptions, staffing ratios, and the
like.

Continuity of care mandates that the plan of care for a
particular patient progresses without interruption. Disruptions
to continuity of care could include such things as missed appointments that are not followed up, tests that are left undone,
X rays that do not get back into the chart on a timely basis,
specific clinical problems that somehow get lost in the shuffle,
consultation or hospitalization that is accomplished without
adequate sharing of information among all providers, and so
forth. Continuity in the ambulatory care setting is not only a
major issue—it is also a major challenge.

The medical record system not only permanently documents
the delivery of care but also serves as an invaluable tool in
actually enhancing the provision of care. The medical record
system provides for timely and accurate recording of all appropriate clinical information so that this information can be easily
tracked and quickly retrieved. Such a system can also provide a
structural framework for evaluating the patient, planning the
treatment course, and delivering health promotion services according to an established program.

Patient risk minimization promotes the concept that it is
important to take all necessary steps to prevent unwanted
change in the patient's health that might result from interaction
with the health care system or organization. Thus, the safety of
the patient while in the facility, infection control, CPR training

for the staff, safety inspections, fire drills, and so forth become quality related issues, since they can distinctly affect the health of the patient. Systems designed to decrease specific *medical* risk to the patient, such as drug profiles and allergy documentation systems, are also important issues here. This area is beginning to receive increasing national attention, generally under the banner of "risk management."

Patient satisfaction assesses the degree to which the health care services and amenities, as well as any resulting changes in health status, meet the expectations of the patient. We are, of course, dealing here with the *perceived* needs of patients; thus, the emphasis is both on providing all required services and on delivering them in such a way that the patient leaves the encounter feeling satisfied. A major focus within this parameter is the "art of care," as delivered not only by the physician but also by the entire ambulatory care organization staff.

Patient compliance is the degree to which the patient accepts and carries out the health care plan developed jointly by the provider and the patient. It is built upon the concept that patients should be active stewards of their own health, and they should therefore share a portion of the responsibility for their own well-being. Patient compliance is also in large part an "art of care" issue; it addresses *relationships* that promote trust and the sharing of information between providers and patients. Patient compliance is a significant quality related parameter because most individualized health care plans simply will not work to best effect without the cooperation of the patient.

Accessibility relates to the ease and timeliness with which health care services can be obtained in the face of such potential barriers as financial, geographical, organizational, emotional, and cultural constraints. A quality organization will clearly make required services available to all patients, at the time these services are most needed. Access to care includes such components as the systematic dissemination of information regarding how to obtain care (sometimes called "outreach"), as well as the ease and timeliness of access both to appointments and to general professional advice (as, for example, on what to do about pain or fever).

Appropriateness of service deals with the fundamental quality issue of whether or not a service, delivered either by the organization as a whole or by a specific provider, is actually indicated in the care of the patient. Inappropriate services (either overtreatment or undertreatment) preclude optimal use of resources in bettering the health status of a total population. Thus, this parameter clearly has both quality and cost implications, and therefore frequently receives major emphasis in proprietary centers. A service may be judged appropriate if it has the real potential to make a positive impact on the health of the patient, and if that potential impact is in some way equivalent to the cost or risk of the service delivered. Of particular importance within this parameter is the appropriateness of diagnostic procedures, medications, and various treatment modalities.

Cost of services recognizes that financial considerations can pose a significant barrier for patients and can therefore have a negative impact on health status. But cost can also have an unwanted impact on quality if the organization, because of cost considerations, can no longer make needed services available. In general, a continuing emphasis should be placed on the reasonableness, fairness, and affordability of the services in question.

It is time now to refer back to the functional definition of quality proposed earlier. You will recall that this definition, put forward by the Institute of Medicine, formed the basis for designating five "dimensions" of quality (as initially identified by Heather Palmer): effectiveness, efficiency, accessibility, acceptability, and provider competence. We can now make a cogent observation regarding our parameters: each relates directly to at least one of the five dimensions, and each thus has a critical interface with the quality of care delivered in an ambulatory care program. (The primary relationship between each parameter and one of the five dimensions is displayed graphically in Figure 9.)

Before leaving our discussion of parameters, we need to note one salient point. At the end of the classic novel *Animal Farm* (Orwell, 1946), a huge sign on the end of the barn wall proclaimed, "ALL ANIMALS ARE EQUAL BUT SOME ANIMALS

**Figure 9. AmbuQual Parameters and Corresponding
Dimensions of Quality.**

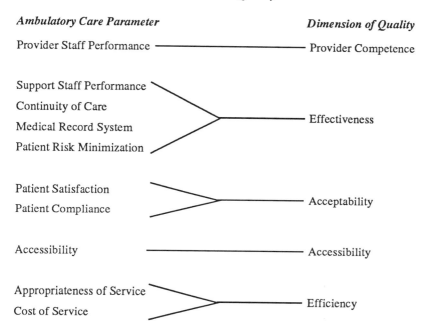

Ambulatory Care Parameter   *Dimension of Quality*

Provider Staff Performance ———————————— Provider Competence

Support Staff Performance
Continuity of Care
Medical Record System   Effectiveness
Patient Risk Minimization

Patient Satisfaction
Patient Compliance   Acceptability

Accessibility   ———————————— Accessibility

Appropriateness of Service
Cost of Service   Efficiency

ARE MORE EQUAL THAN OTHERS." The same is true in the
Quality Assurance barnyard. Donabedian (1987, p. 27) has written, "[It] seems self-evident that the criteria cannot be of equal
importance; failure to comply with some should have more
serious consequences than failure to abide by others." We con-
cur, and we have addressed this issue by developing a weighting
system that factors in the relative impact on health status for any
given indicator. This system flows through all of AmbuQual, and
it forms one of the foundations of the overall scoring system. Its
first application is in the parameters we have just described.
Each parameter receives a different scoring weight, based on its
relative impact on patient health. The average of all parameter
weights is 1.0.

This weighting scale is not arbitrary; it is, rather, the
product of substantial investigation and research. We surveyed

fifty ambulatory care surveyors from the Joint Commission, asking them to compare each of the parameters with every other parameter (a paired comparison exercise involving forty-five separate pairings). Forty-eight of the surveyors responded; twenty were administrators, and the remainder were various primary care and specialty physicians. The responses were then put through several different statistical models to ensure their overall validity. According to a research document produced by personnel from Purdue University and Methodist Hospital of Indiana (Anderson and others, 1988, pp. 2, 5), "The results suggest that the ten weighted parameters provide a sensitive measure of professional perceptions of the relative impact of ambulatory care activities on the health of ambulatory patients. . . . The ten ambulatory care parameters are behaviorally based measures of quality of care that would have a direct effect on a patient's health." These study results indicate that each parameter does, indeed, measure a single dimension of perceived quality, and that they are additive. The same researchers also concluded that "there was a high level of agreement among the 48 judges," regardless of the career group they represented.

As we might have predicted, provider staff performance was judged the most important of the ten parameters in determining health outcomes. Thus, it received the highest scoring weight—nearly four times that of cost (which, perhaps surprisingly, was determined to have the least perceived impact on the health status of the patient). The final weightings now used in the AmbuQual system are as follows:

Provider staff performance = 1.92
Appropriateness of service = 1.39
Patient compliance   = 1.25
Support staff performance = 1.11
Accessibility   = .91
Continuity of care   = .90
Patient risk minimization = .70
Medical record system   = .68
Patient satisfaction   = .59
Cost of services   = .54

Aspects of Care. With these parameters as the starting point, we next developed specific aspects of care for each parameter. While as a practical matter many of our selected aspects represent processes, systems, and so forth that are (in JCAHO's words) "high-volume, high-risk, or problem-prone," this was not the determining factor in the aspects' selection; rather, they were chosen as logical subdivisions of our parameters. Each of the ten parameters has been divided into four aspects, for a total of forty; a good sample of these aspects is displayed in Resource C, under the parameters to which they relate.

In selecting the specific aspects for each of the parameters, we also asked ourselves one basic question: "Does this aspect truly affect the health of the patient?" Notice that we did not begin by asking ourselves, "Does this aspect improve the care given to the patient?" The first question ultimately leads to a broader, more outcome related orientation.

The sample aspects in Resource C also show that our use of weighting scales for input into the overall scoring system does not end with parameters. Thus, each aspect has also been weighted, according to our perception of its relative impact on the health of the patient. Within the parameter of provider staff performance, for example, the aspect of "credentials" is believed to be two times as important in impacting the health of the patient as the aspect of "provider staff systems," but it is not considered to have as much impact as "clinical performance." Within each parameter, the average weight of all aspects is 1.0.

Indicators of Quality. Armed with a total of forty aspects of care, the next step was development of specific indicators of quality for each aspect. No such formalized theory as for aspect selection was used in choosing indicators; the real objective was to essentially "cover the waterfront" by specifying all significant factors within any single aspect. Thus, one aspect may have two indicators that relate to it, while another may include six or seven. In all, AmbuQual addresses roughly 150 indicators.

Sample indicators (grouped within their appropriate aspects) are also shown in Resource C. Some, we believe, apply equally well to virtually all ambulatory care organizations; these are marked with an asterisk in Resource C. However, the possible organizational variations in size, form, complexity, purpose, and so on that are possible in the ambulatory care field preclude one set of indicators being fully applicable everywhere; therefore, the nonasterisked indicators are those that have been chosen specifically for HealthNet, and for which locally generated indicators specific to any given organization could easily be substituted.

For each indicator, an appropriate criterion and related standard have been specifically delineated. Thus, as an example, an indicator entitled "support staff" (under the aspect titled "satisfaction with staff," which is part of the patient satisfaction parameter) has as its criterion, "Patients indicate satisfaction with the support staff." The standard [known in AmbuQual as a "quality improvement plan (QIP) level"] has been organizationally set at 80 percent; thus, any score below 80 on the evaluation of this indicator will result in corrective action (or at the least, further in-depth analysis).

Each indicator also includes a specified data source. The indicator for "support staff" derives its input, for instance, from our formal "Give Us a Grade" patient satisfaction audit; specifically, three questions on this audit provide explicit patient generated data on the courtesy and perceived competence of various support staff categories. Other data sources include our routine performance audit and procedure audit (both noted previously), various written policies, documented procedures, and formal verification systems for provider and support staff credentialing.

Finally, each indicator is assigned a responsibility focal point; this is the person or position assigned the responsibility (and authority) to correct any identified problems or to pursue any specified improvements related to this indicator. Thus, since both the organizational standard and the specific focus of responsibility are fixed well before actual evaluation begins, the assignment of subsequent problems and opportunities can be perceived as impersonal.

Once all of the components of the system were developed, we initiated a schedule for Quality Assurance committee review

Figure 10. Sample Indicator.

INDICATOR: "Medication Sensitivity Documentation"

>   Criterion: All medicine sensitivities must be clearly
>   documented according to the organization's
>   specific plan for such activity.
>   Standard ("QIP Level"): 70
>   Data Source: Performance Audit (Question #25)
>   Weight: 1.1
>   Scoring: Quantitative (Computer)
>   Responsibility: Medical Director

of all indicators (and thus all aspects and parameters). In addition, the concept of a "generic indicators chart" was developed; this is an integrated chart of all components of the AmbuQual system, arrayed by specific indicator and related elements. These indicators are grouped into the appropriate aspects, and the aspects are subsequently grouped into the respective parameters. Figure 10 gives an example of one entry from the generic indicators chart.

Through this mechanism, Quality Assurance activity can be easily and quickly understood and routinely applied.

Scoring. There are actually two scoring processes involved in the application of AmbuQual. The first, which is the essence of the Quality Assurance committee's routine function, is the regular evaluation (by specific indicator) that results from ongoing monitoring through the generic indicators chart noted above. The second is the aggregation, at several levels, of all related scores that flow from this Quality Assurance committee activity.

The committee's scoring process revolves around whether the indicator in question is listed as "Quantitative" (as in the example above) or "Qualitative." As Chapter Seven also described, a quantitative indicator (which falls into the category of assessment carried out through "explicit" criteria/standards sets) is one for which an absolute number flows automatically from the data source, as in the case of a summarization of patient responses to a specific patient satisfaction question. The committee's task for this type of indicator is simply to ensure that the numerical value is being produced by the data source as required, and to report this number to the total organization via Quality Assurance committee meeting minutes.

A qualitative indicator, on the other hand, is one for which the listed data source produces no hard numerical value. Thus, this type of assessment generally relies on implicit criteria. A good example would be evaluation of whether or not a certain procedure (for instance, lab quality control) is accurate, up to date, functional, and appropriately utilized. In order to assess such an indicator, the Quality Assurance committee must discuss, deliberate, vote, and ultimately reach a consensus regarding the level of performance relative to the organizational standard.

Each such indicator is assigned a presenter, a member of the Quality Assurance committee who has the task of researching the issue based on the wording of the specific criterion and then reporting the findings to the full committee. Follow-up discussion is held until all questions regarding the organizational performance and its impact on patient care have been sufficiently answered. The committee then votes individually on the level of performance regarding the indicator. The form utilized is shown as Exhibit 3; a companion "key" allows each vote to be translated into numerical equivalents for both "standard fulfillment" and "probable impact," with a total possible score of 100. (The double boxes for each scoring level give the option of scoring through a two-vote mechanism, in which the sequential votes allow members to adjust their final evaluations based on ideas gained from ongoing open group discussion.)

Both halves of the voting form are completed by each committee member, and the scores are averaged for both "standard fulfillment" and "probable impact of deficiencies on patient care." The two resulting scores are then added to produce the final score, which equates to a percentage (since the highest

**Exhibit 3. AmbuQual Evaluation Scoring Form
(for Qualitative Indicators Only).**

Qualitative Scoring	
Indicator #: _____	Initials: _____
Standard Fulfillment	**Probable Impact of Deficiencies on Patient Care**
☐ ☐ Completely fulfilled.	☐ ☐ No deficiencies.
☐ ☐ Nearly fulfilled.	☐ ☐ Minimal impact: "Paper or technical requirement."
☐ ☐ More than half fulfilled.	☐ ☐ Moderate impact: "Should be improved."
☐ ☐ Half fulfilled.	
☐ ☐ Less than half fulfilled.	☐ ☐ Significant impact: "Worrisome; important omissions."
☐ ☐ Barely fulfilled.	☐ ☐ Critical impact: "Urgent; must be promptly corrected; severe compromise."
☐ ☐ Not fulfilled at all.	• Automatic zero if standard is not fulfilled at all.

possible total score for both issues is 100). If required, a corrective action mandate is then issued, as discussed below.

At this point, the second scoring mechanism is called into play. Once a given indicator has been scored (by either the quantitative or qualitative method), it is added to the scores of all other indicators that compose the "parent" aspect of care. That aspect's overall score is then aggregated with the scores of the other three aspects to develop an overall score for the respective parameter. Finally, scores for all of the ten parameters are added together to develop the ultimate organizational score, known as the Program Quality Index (or "PQI"). A diagram showing the flow of this scoring system for the sample parameter of "patient risk minimization" (without actual scores or weights) is shown in Figure 11. This system effectively represents a hierarchy of scores that feed upward until a single index of quality for the total organization is achieved, as Figure 12 graphically displays. Of course, all appropriate weights are factored in at each successive step; the final result then becomes a set of numbers that indicates the current level of quantified "quality," both for the organization as a whole and for each of its component parts. These numbers can be tracked by computer to provide an instantaneous readout of the current quality level. We compute all numbers on a monthly basis, and produce a line graph to indicate quality trends over time. Thus, as the following chapter will further describe, AmbuQual can be a powerful instrument not only for measuring quality, but also for actively managing it.

Specifying Corrective Action. Every time an indicator falls below the score established by the related organizational standard, the Quality Assurance committee generates what is known as a quality improvement plan (or "QIP"). A completed QIP form is displayed in Chapter Ten. This instrument is a simple yet powerful tool that provides significant help in processing both basic Quality Assurance information and mandates regarding necessary corrective action. This form integrates all information required in the assigning, tracking, and resolving of identified problems or opportunities to improve. It also allows the Quality Assurance committee to prioritize ongoing Quality Assurance efforts within the organization, and it helps provide the "clout factor" needed to ensure that corrective action is taken (and is ultimately successful in solving identified problems).

As one can see on the completed QIP form in Chapter Ten, this instrument shows precisely what the problem is, which manager is responsible for solving it, where the related indicator can be found in AmbuQual, how the Quality Assurance committee scored the indicator (that is, what the magnitude of the problem appears to be), and what issues should be considered in solving the problem. (This recommendations section is optional, since, as has been established, the Quality Assurance committee does not have the job of actually solving the problem, but simply points it out and tracks it to resolution.)

The QIP form also requires the Quality Assurance com-

Figure 11. The AmbuQual System: "Patient Risk Minimization" Example.

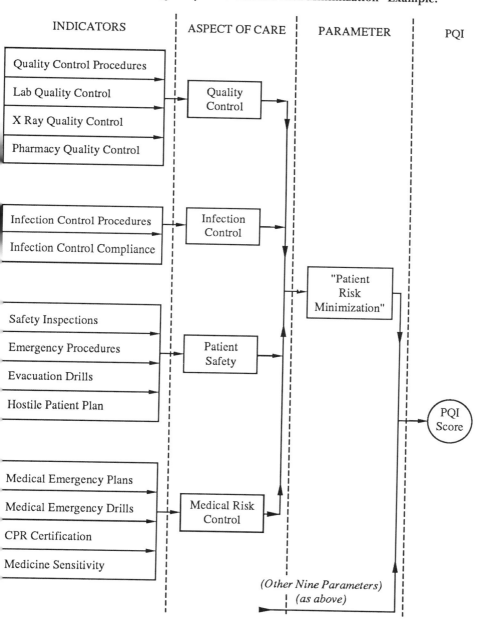

Figure 12. AmbuQual Evaluation and Scoring Flow.

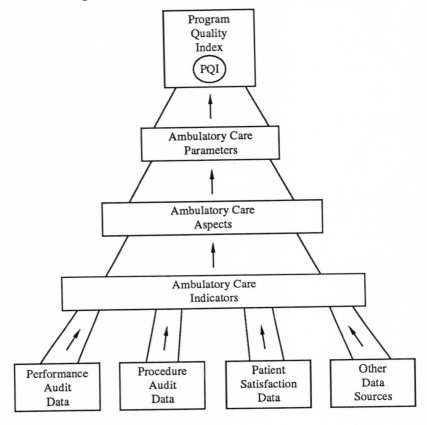

mittee to assign a target date for resolution of the problem. This is essentially for setting priorities. If, for example, the committee feels that the problem is significant and has a serious potential impact on patient care and resulting health status, a tight deadline can be imposed. Normally, however, a deadline of three to six months is assigned.

The QIP form also documents final resolution of the problem; this feature helps provide organizational "clout" to the Quality Assurance effort and thus fosters active problem solving. During the month following the deadline set for problem resolution, the committee again scores the indicator in question, largely as if it were assigning an initial score. Notice that the committee does *not* simply judge the intervening action taken on the problem, although a discussion of this action might be part of the committee's rescoring process. The philosophy at work here is that the *results*, rather than the specific corrective actions, are most important. Thus, the most recent status of the indicator itself should be the benchmark by which the effectiveness of problem solving should be judged.

If, at the time of this rescoring process, the Quality Assurance committee finds that the standard is still not met (and, therefore, that the original problem still exists), it produces a "director's QIP." This is sent (on red paper, no less) to the organization's executive director, and it then becomes that person's responsibility to ensure that the problem is solved. Of course, it is probable that the director will simply take action to find out why the manager to whom the QIP was originally sent did not succeed in solving the problem. And if the director is also unable to effect resolution (as documented by still further Quality Assurance committee review of the indicator), the QIP then becomes a "governing body QIP." Since the governing body has hiring and termination authority over the director, and the director in turn has the same authority over all of the organization's managers, it is clear how the "clout factor" is assured through this system.

The QIP form, then, moves the corrective action system, while the generic indicators chart drives the routine Quality Assurance committee process. The combined result is the overall AmbuQual program, a system that produces quantitative judgments about quality within both the total entity and the individual organizational components. Public display of quantifiable improvement (or lack thereof) serves to significantly invest the staff in the ongoing assessment process, as accomplished through the multidisciplinary Quality Assurance committee.

AmbuQual thus enables a structured, ongoing, and comprehensive look at the total quality of care within the organization. AmbuQual employs prospective and explicit criteria and standards for both clinical and organizational indicators, and it enables subjective input as needed through the qualitative scoring process.

This system has now been field tested and shown to be highly replicable; additionally, it can be easily adapted to virtually any ambulatory care program, regardless of size or type. In short, we believe it provides an integrated, unified, and valid instrument for the ongoing assessment—and ultimately, management—of quality of care in the ambulatory care setting.

Chapter 10

Resolving Problems and Tracking Results

It is expensive to be mediocre in this world. . . . Quality is always cost-effective.

> —J. Irwin Miller, Cummins
> Engine Company

If monitoring and evaluation identifies a potential quality related problem or significant opportunity for quality improvement, the problem resolution phase of the two-phase Quality Assurance process is activated. Thus, Step Seven in our generic model is the accomplishment of appropriate action when the organization's standards have not been met, and Step Eight is evaluation of the ultimate effect of this action.

When a discrepancy exists between expected and actual performance, immediate remedial action will clearly be needed in some instances; in other cases, the most appropriate action might well be more intensive evaluation (often by professional personnel) to determine whether or not a justifiable variance has occurred. When corrective action is undertaken, it is a sound idea to track "resolved" problems for up to several years, since deficiencies have a disturbing tendency to recur. (Of course, if monitoring is routine and periodic from the outset, any tendency to backslide should be caught automatically.)

Basic Problem-Solving Issues

Corrective action cannot be random if it is to be successful. Crosby (1979, p. 26) says regarding problems that "the lack of a disciplined method of openly attacking them breeds more problems." In order to preclude this, the Quality Assurance committee must answer four important questions for the organization (and especially for those responsible for solving problems).

What Is the Exact Nature of the Problem? At the outset, the Quality Assurance committee must precisely specify the nature of the problem for the organization. Some discrepancies, of course, may not be as worthwhile to pursue as others; therefore, the committee must be able to separate the wheat from the chaff. Two questions can help in this endeavor.

First, can the problem really be solved? Some deficiencies are so firmly rooted in permanent structures, ongoing issues, or lack of needed resources that the likelihood of real resolution may, at least initially, be rather slim; thus, valuable time should not be spent on insoluble problems. However, the Quality Assurance process can perform an invaluable service by highlighting these problems for the organization's ultimate decision makers, who must then determine if such problems are, in fact, important enough to justify the requisite organizational trade-offs (such as transferring available resources from other projects).

Second, is the benefit (primarily to the patient, but also to the organization itself) actually worth the cost (in all forms) of attempting to solve the problem? The operative thought here: Don't spend a dollar on a dime problem.

Who Should Solve the Problem? AmbuQual, for example, prospectively specifies on the generic indicators chart (as well as directly on the QIP form) which manager is to be tasked with problem resolution for each indicator. This does not always need to be specified in advance, however, to be effective; it can often simply be done when problems are identified. Houser says that in his program, "there are no predetermined problem solvers — we simply assign the responsibility when we note the problem, according to what the deficiency is."

Of course, the Quality Assurance committee's ultimate

answer regarding who will solve the problem is "someone else." One of the earliest principles discussed in this book was that the Quality Assurance committee does not actually solve deficiencies; this is a management responsibility, and throwing another entity into the pot badly blurs organizational lines of authority and responsibility. Sometimes it is difficult for the committee to avoid jumping in; as Biller says, "It takes a leap of faith not to let the committee actually *do* Quality Assurance." This must, however, be avoided.

It will be worthwhile in this context to briefly revisit our earlier discussion (from Chapter Five) of the actual role of the Quality Assurance committee, specifically with reference to this issue of problem solving.

All of our five study programs in some fashion cause the initiation of specific corrective action to occur at the lowest possible level within the organization; that is, problem solving is essentially decentralized. This decentralization is actively mandated, for instance, through the documented Quality Assurance philosophies (as found in the respective Quality Assurance plans) underlying the total programs in Cambridge and Indianapolis.

In Fremont, decentralization of problem solving flows in large part from the small size of the organization itself, the general physical and emotional closeness of the staff, and the relative informality of day-to-day processes; all of these as a practical matter foster an environment in which problems are frequently resolved "on the spot" and simply reported (after the fact) to the Quality Assurance committee. (It should be noted, however, that the Quality Assurance committee does occasionally direct specific corrective action if it is clear that problem solving has failed at lower levels.)

It is in the two programs undergoing the most active transition — those in Atlanta and Chicago — where the decentralization of problem solving responsibility is even remotely at issue. In practice, corrective action at the lowest level is the norm in these two programs; however, largely as a function of the increasing emphasis on, and integration of, Quality Assurance as a major organizational process, the Quality Assurance committee at each site can itself take a role at some point in the problem-solving activity.

Winer states that in the Chicago program, "one of our current intentions is to assemble a more autonomous, integrated Quality Assurance program from the component pieces that have traditionally existed. This will also involve some increasing centralization of Quality Assurance effort." Thus, while specific ambulatory care clinics perform the actual monitoring and evaluation of their areas (and take first-line corrective action whenever appropriate), their task is to report monitoring results through the rather complex Quality Assurance structure described in both Chapter Three and Resource A. Much of the corrective action is then either directed by or taken at these successive levels.

In the Atlanta program, as the total Quality Assurance process becomes more overtly formalized, it is also becoming more centralized. As Mary Driscoll, director of quality control for Southeastern Health Services, says, "With increasing sophistication and greater formality in our systems, we'll need to be actively on our guard to ensure that the Quality Assurance process doesn't lose the constant touch with lower levels that we now have." In its current configuration, the Quality Assurance committee can, in fact, take an active hand in the problem-solving process if desired. As a practical matter, however, this happens relatively infrequently.

Do either of these processes really work in day-to-day practice? That is, does either the strict decentralization of problem-solving responsibility or the activation of a hierarchy of responsibility levels allow significant problems to go unaddressed? The evidence is that there are, in fact, very few "holes" in any of the processes in place at the five study sites. For example, Winer remarks that in the Chicago system, "we rarely see anything fall through the cracks. There are usually several simultaneous looks at any given issue, and my department serves as the coordinating link throughout the entire system." In the Fremont program, says Cockerline, "we really feel that we do improve quality, and our staff sees Quality Assurance as one of the best available means to solve their own problems." And in

Cambridge, Biller says, "Someone once said that trying to sneak a pitch past Hank Aaron was like trying to sneak the sunrise past a rooster. . . . Around here, the committee and I together are Hank Aaron."

What Will Be Considered Sufficient Resolution of the Problem? The answer here is simply, whatever the Quality Assurance committee will accept as evidence that the deficiency has been corrected. This can be decided by reviewing either the action itself or the results of that action. The AmbuQual system, as noted in the previous chapter, simply rescores the indicator; that is, results alone are assessed. Other programs look at corrective actions. Either approach can work; however, if the corrective action itself is reviewed, the organization must somehow also ensure that the originating problem is actually solved by this action.

In either case, the Quality Assurance committee must have the decision-making authority. Note that this does not preclude another person or group — the executive director or the governing body, for example — from deciding that even though the problem still exists, it is not worth the organizational effort and expense to go any further in trying to fix it. Nor does it keep another person or group from suggesting that, although the committee has judged a problem to be resolved, some vestiges of the problem may still exist. Nevertheless, it is the committee's ultimate authority to judge when a problem has *not* been fully resolved. And in practice, such a decision may often necessitate calling on the "clout factor" that must be organizationally built into Quality Assurance, to enable problems remaining unresolved (in the committee's view) to be immediately pushed up to a higher organizational level. As we have seen, each of our five studied programs has developed a structure that enables this to occur whenever required.

Of course, one possibility is that further evaluation of the problem itself will be necessary. Here again, the two programs in active transition (Atlanta and Chicago) are the most likely to task the Quality Assurance committee itself with performing this further study; the other three programs use the committee primarily to push the task of detailed evaluation back down into the operational environment. (It should also be noted, however, that in Atlanta and Chicago the Quality Assurance committees are likely to direct the full-time—and in both cases relatively large—Quality Assurance professional staffs to either perform or actively facilitate any required additional study.)

What Is the Target Date by Which the Problem Should Be Resolved?
The Quality Assurance committee must establish appropriate target dates. Through this process, the committee can set priorities for the quality related problems with which the organization must deal. Deadlines should not be set too far into the future, of course; the programs we visited (most notably the Washington Outpatient Surgery Center, where daily resolution is the expected norm) generally wanted to give problems speedy attention. However, especially if an issue is complex or needs further study, an overly ambitious target date could easily be counterproductive. For this reason, we found quarterly review of assigned corrective action to be a frequently specified time frame.

Solving Problems by Changing Performance

When a problem has been identified, the organization will commonly use several conventional avenues to solve it, including modifying systems (procedures, structures, and so forth); improving documentation; strengthening data collection; providing more training; developing motivational techniques and instituting incentive systems; and, generally as a last resort, implementing disciplinary action. The only change that will truly make any long-term difference in the health status of the patient, however, is a change in human or organizational performance.

A good example of this notion has already been mentioned in another context. At HealthNet, a special study showed us that a surprising number of patients with hypertension were not sufficiently controlled by the treatments being prescribed. In fact, in-service training had been held, continuing education sessions had been attended, and the problem of hypertension management had been given substantial emphasis in meetings; that is, physicians had, indeed, improved their *knowledge* of hypertension therapies, but they were still being less than optimally effective in reducing actual hypertension readings. This effect is a common one (due to the complexity of hypertension itself, various patient compliance issues, and so forth), and other methods have since been devised to help address the problem; the point here is simply that taking an immediate and obvious action (such as providing more educational opportunities) does not of itself guarantee that performance will actually be changed.

An effective Quality Assurance program must, therefore, routinely track corrective action results over time until it is clear that the originating problem has been fully resolved through a true change in human/organizational performance. Each of our five model programs has successfully dealt with this issue; a few cogent examples will help make this point.

The Washington Outpatient Surgery Center identified a problem involving patients who were arriving for surgery out of compliance with appropriate NPO status (that is, having taken food or drink after a specified cutoff time). Expectations were then clarified with physicians, and patients themselves received pre-op phone calls. Continued problem tracking, however, indicated that a problem still clearly existed; as a result, even more intensive physician education was undertaken. Subsequent follow-up monitoring was then performed a year after the problem was first detected, and the noted result was "very low incidence of patients not NPO — problem resolved." Yet another reevaluation six months later indicated that ongoing performance had, indeed, been improved, and that the problem remained resolved; nevertheless, constant reevaluation continues to assure nonrecurrence.

In Chicago, an increased emphasis on immunization rates in the general pediatrics clinics improved overall variance levels for these clinics by a range of 11–17 percent, as validated by restudy of the original problem. Clearly, performance had been changed for the better.

We have discussed the documented decrease in the repeat film rate in Cambridge to well below the national average. Clearly the Quality Assurance process has facilitated (and continually confirmed) a positive change in performance. Also at this site, the addition of personnel in the dermatology and ear, nose, and throat (ENT) clinics was later found to have been successful in reducing long waiting times; organizational performance had been verifiably improved.

In sum, while all of the programs have used Quality Assurance to make needed changes in systems, procedures, education, and so forth, the more important issue is that actual results have borne out real changes in individual and organizational performance. This is the true "bottom line" for Quality Assurance.

A final note is needed here on one specific avenue to verifiably changing provider performance. This is the idea of rewarding providers based upon the quality of the care they render, as documented in part through the Quality Assurance process. Here, again, Ernest Codman was a true visionary; in 1914, he stated his belief (then thought eccentric) that health care organizations "must promote members of the staff on a basis which gives due consideration to what they . . . accomplish for their patients." The reverse of promotion is, of course, professional sanctions. Both of these mechanisms for change, based at least partly on Quality Assurance findings, can be seen at work in our studied programs.

In the HealthNet system, for instance, we have recently instituted a provider compensation package including, among other things, structured incentives for documented quality of care. Our program also requires specific, ongoing documentation regarding credentialing and privileging.

In Atlanta, the Quality Assurance program helps provide information that can, if significant enough, be used to deny partnership in the group and to withhold practice privileges.

Specific attention to both initial and recurrent privileging is also found (in differing forms, depending upon the specific institution) in the programs in Cambridge, Chicago, and Fremont.

This is one of the waves of the future. We believe that the use of financial rewards and privileging sanctions, initiated largely through Quality Assurance activity, will increase. We also believe this is necessary if Quality Assurance is to function effectively in improving actual performance.

Tracking Program Results

Problem solving is initially an immediate activity; as problems are identified, problem solving kicks in until the deficiency is resolved. However, as noted, the same problems can too easily return. Thus, a mechanism for tracking at least certain issues over time is a prerequisite for a strong Quality Assurance program. Even better is any mechanism for routinely following the trend of an entire program, to ensure ongoing improvement in total program quality; it is at this point that Quality Assurance begins to approach Quality Management.

Actually, general trust in the long-term salutary effects of Quality Assurance is at present as much a matter of faith as of fact; however, we continue to believe that a valid assessment and problem-solving process will allow us to steadily "notch up," in stairstep fashion, our organization's quality level year by year. While this is still basically unproven, we at least know that quality improvement through problem solving will not come overnight. As one writer (Perry, 1981, p. 51) has put it, "Developing a quality environment. . . is a long-range program."

In spite of the long-term nature of real change, we must make the leap of faith. The Center for Disease Control suggests that 20,000 people die each year as the direct result of nosocomial (hospital-acquired) infections; here is a clear example of the real need to solve important clinical problems, and we believe Quality Assurance is the appropriate vehicle for addressing such issues. But to truly validate the benefits of this process, we must be able to document that such problems are solved and remain solved.

All of our five programs have developed specific formats to track program results. Some systems, as in Atlanta, are tracked primarily through ongoing reports and meeting minutes. Others, such as the Cambridge program, have developed explicit forms that facilitate continual tracking of the current status of problems and corrective actions for all monitored indicators. And some, such as the programs in Indianapolis and Chicago, either have or will soon implement computerized capabilities for continually tracking Quality Assurance problem resolution activities, as well as overall program results.

Perhaps most exciting is the potential for real quality *management* through documented problem solving and routine tracking of related results. One powerful example can be found in the current capabilities of the computerized AmbuQual system. Tables 1 and 2 and Exhibit 4 will walk the reader through a real-life issue recently addressed by the Quality Assurance committee and HealthNet's management, as described below.

The overall program quality index (PQI) for HealthNet had dropped by several points over the course of four months, from 78 to 74. A look at the PQI table (Table 1) shows that while most parameter scores had either remained constant or had improved slightly, the score for provider staff performance had declined by 20 points. The related aspect comparison table (Table 2) for all four aspects within the parameter indicates that "current competence" had declined precipitously during the four-month period, from 75 to 16. Within this aspect (which substantially deals with issues of documentation), the specific indicator for "health status" had declined from 100 to 31, while the indicator for "review of privileges" had dropped to 0 (from a previous score of 100).

Both of these indicators, as it happens, had recently received a QIP (a corrective action mandate) from the Quality Assurance committee; the QIP for "review of privileges" is shown as Exhibit 4. Since the weight— the organization's perception of relative impact on patient health status— of the indicator dealing with privileges is fully 300 percent of the weight for "health status," a shrewd manager would, if resources were at all limited, place these resources first at the disposal of the person responsible for solving the "review of privileges" issue.

This was, in the final analysis, a structural/documentation problem, rather than a first-line quality of care problem; the

Table 1. Sample PQI Table.

8/28/88 Neighborhood Health Centers			Score				
Parameter	Description	Weight	Apr.	May	June	July	Aug.
1	Provider Staff Performance	1.92	81	81	76	61	61
2	Support Staff Performance	1.11	86	85	84	85	84
3	Continuity of Care	.90	69	71	71	72	72
4	Medical Record System	.68	83	82	81	81	81
5	Patient Risk Minimization	.70	64	66	65	64	64
6	Patient Satisfaction	.59	88	90	91	90	91
7	Patient Compliance	1.25	73	74	75	76	76
8	Accessibility	.91	86	85	87	86	86
9	Appropriateness of Service	1.39	63	64	62	63	63
10	Cost of Service	.54	87	87	87	87	87
PROGRAM QUALITY INDEX			78	78	76	74	74

issue was resolved once privileging documentation was updated. However, had the issue been one of a functional provider performance deficiency, the potential impact on quality of care could obviously have been significant. In any case, AmbuQual was able to facilitate actual quality management by pointing out and defining a precise problem, assigning resources to solve the problem, and actively prioritizing those assigned resources. Once the problem was completely resolved and the indicator was rescored, the resulting quantitative index for the indicator in question reflected problem resolution. This indicator score then took its place among other aggregated indicator/aspect scores to demonstrate improvement in the quantified status of quality for our organization as a whole.

The monitoring and evaluation process thus leads to problem solving, and ultimately to program quality improve-

Table 2. Sample Aspect Comparison Table.

Neighborhood Health Centers			Score	
	Description	Weight	Apr.	Aug.
Parameter 1	Provider Staff Performance	1.92	81	61
Aspect A	Credentials	1.00	87	69
1.A.1	Educational background	1.00	89	79
1.A.2	Training	1.00	89	89
1.A.3	Experience	1.25	90	0
1.A.4	Certification	1.25	75	100
1.A.5	Licensure	.50	100	100
Aspect B	Provider Staff Systems	.50	87	83
1.B.1	Job descriptions	1.00	79	90
1.B.2	Policies and procedures	1.00	96	95
1.B.3	Personnel perf. eval. — systems	1.00	99	100
1.B.4	Continuing ed. — policy	1.00	79	25
1.B.5	Peer review audit syst.	1.00	93	100
1.B.6	Provider staff protocols	1.00	74	85
Aspect C	**Current Competence**	1.00	**75**	**16**
1.C.1	Health status	.50	**100**	**31**
1.C.2	**Review of privileges**	1.50	**100**	**0**
1.C.3	CE — Units earned	1.00	0	0
1.C.4	Personnel perf. eval. — result	1.00	100	50
Aspect D	Clinical Performance	1.50	76	78
1.D.1	General clinical performance audit	1.50	93	93
1.D.2	Health outcome audits	1.00	67	67
1.D.3	Policies and procedures — utilized	1.00	80	80
1.D.4	Whole person perf. audit	1.00	85	85
1.D.5	Health maint. perf. audit	1.00	64	64
1.D.6	Prob. focused clin. study	.50	0	25
1.D.7	Clin. indicators audit	1.00	99	99

ment — or at least we all trust that is so. But the ultimate goal for Quality Assurance is to move beyond the point at which we have to *solve* problems to a time in which we can actively *prevent* them; while this may not be likely for some time, it is nonetheless an eminently worthy goal. As Crosby (1984, p. 67) says, "What has to happen is *prevention*. The error that does not exist cannot be missed."

Exhibit 4. Sample AmbuQual Quality Improvement Plan.

1. <u>Neighborhood Health Centers</u>   Date <u>8</u> / <u>17</u> / <u>88</u>   QIP# <u>131</u>
    Name of Organization/Dept/Division   Assigned   (optional)

2. <u>William Van Osdel, M.D.</u>   <u>Prof. Staff Coordinator</u>
    Manager Responsible for QIP   Job Title

3. QIP Description for Computerized Log:

`R e v i e w   o f   P r o v i d e r   P r i v i l e g e s   C u r r e n t`

                 (Description can be no longer than 40 characters long)

4. QIP Narrative Description (reason for QIP)

    <u>According to the schedule established by Management, "privilege"</u>
    <u>documentation for providers expired 6/88.</u>

5. Related AMBUQUAL Indicator # <u>1C2</u> , Standard: <u>"All providers must be currently</u>
    <u>privileged (by the Governing Body) for all procedures performed."</u>

6. Indicator Score <u>0</u>   Related QIP Level (threshold) <u>70%</u>

7. QA Committee's Recommendations for QIP Resolution (optional) <u>Seek Board approval of all provider</u>
    <u>privileges by assigned target date (below). Provide final</u>
    <u>documentation.</u>

8. Target Date for Resolution <u>11</u> / <u>30</u> / <u>88</u>   X <u>_Peyton Towne, J._</u>
                                      (QA Committee Chair's Signature)

---

9. RESOLUTION

Review Date ___ / ___ / ___   Indicator Score _____   Above QIP Level = Resolved _____

                                At/ Below QIP Level = Director's QIP _____

Director's QIP
Review Date ___ / ___ / ___   Indicator Score _____   Above QIP Level = Resolved _____

                                At/ Below QIP Level = Governing Body's QIP _____

Governing Body QIP Decision _____

Review Date ___ / ___ / ___

           X _____
                   (QA Committee Chair's Signature)

---

10. Distribution:
     1) Copy to Manager Responsible
     2) Copy to Head of Initiating Organization, Department or Division
     3) Original and copy of all updates to QA Document File

Chapter 11

*Formalizing Quality Assurance
Through a Written Record*

No one likes to document. . . . This doesn't mean we are
bad people — only that we are like everyone else.
— William E. Perry,
*Hatching the EDP Quality
Assurance Function*

A time-honored organizational maxim suggests, "If it isn't documented, it isn't done." Quality Assurance, like every other component of organizational life, falls under the purview of this
bureaucratic truism. While documentation may not be at the
top of everyone's list of favorite activities, it is nonetheless vital to
the long-term effectiveness of quality assessment. As Perry (1981,
p. 49) put it, "Unless [documenting is] enforced, the quality
assurance function will have neither the power . . . nor the
tools . . . to carry off [its] function."

A key element in the Quality Assurance plan should be a
requirement for development of appropriate methods to oversee the effectiveness of monitoring and evaluation, as well as a
means to validate problem-solving activity. In order for these
tasks to be fully accomplished, regular documentation of program activities must be generated; furthermore, these documented activities must be routinely reported to all appropriate
parties if needed information is to be truly integrated throughout the organization. These activities constitute the final major
task (Step Nine) in our generic model.

In general, five items should be routinely documented
and reported: findings, conclusions, recommendations, actions
taken, and results of the actions taken. At The University of

172

Chicago Hospitals, the standard documenting/reporting format throughout the entire Quality Assurance program is formally specified by the acronym DCRAE, for Discussion, Conclusions, Recommendations, Actions, and Evaluation. Thus, meetings are routinely structured around this basically sequential format (which directly addresses the issues to be documented and reported), and meeting minutes and resulting reports are put into DCRAE format for both easy standardization and general process facilitation.

The real purposes of a strong documentation and reporting system are to appropriately assign and track corrective actions and effectively weave all quality related information routinely into the operational fabric of the organization. A rigorous documentation/reporting system is especially useful in more complex organizations, such as MIT or The University of Chicago Hospitals. In such entities, Quality Assurance activities and information often cut across departmental or functional lines, and a strong system of documentation can do much both to help spot interdepartmental problems or trends and to encourage appropriate sharing of Quality Assurance responsibilities.

A brief side note is in order on documenting confidentiality of information. The Quality Assurance program will obviously be involved at times with organizational information that should be treated as highly sensitive. Therefore, it is wise to specifically document the organization's policy on release of such information; in some cases, state laws apply. A clear statement of policy regarding confidentiality of Quality Assurance information can be made directly in the Quality Assurance plan, as seen in the plan from the Atlanta program (displayed in Resource E). Or, it can be made via some other document commonly used in the Quality Assurance process; such, for example, is the case at HealthNet, where the QIP form (shown in Chapter Ten) specifically states a confidentiality warning at the bottom.

Documenting the Problem-Solving and Tracking Process

Some Ideas Regarding Format. As we have suggested, one major function of a good documentation system is facilitation of problem solving. To accomplish this, the system must provide a means to sufficiently document problem identification, as well as a mechanism to track actions taken to solve the problem or to pursue a specific opportunity to improve performance. We will look briefly at the systems used in three of our sites as good examples of formal documentation of problem solving.

In Indianapolis, as we have noted, several specific audits produce many of the data for Quality Assurance committee review, and each of these audits utilizes its own specific documentation. As an example, the basic performance audit format (one page of which is shown as Exhibit 5) consists of a number of both general and protocol-specific questions, the answers to which are documented on the audit form itself. A separate performance audit feedback form then documents ongoing follow-up dialogue between the review committee and the physician being evaluated, as well as the ultimate disposition of relevant findings; a final section of this specific form generates special studies, as needed. All of the quarterly audit findings are then summarized, and a quarterly summation report (by specific audit question) is generated. All resulting data feed directly into the AmbuQual system for monitoring by the Quality Assurance committee. As noted in Chapter Nine, this committee then employs a single quality improvement plan (QIP) sheet to assign any needed corrective action and to track the originating problem to full resolution. All documentation resulting from these activities feeds into the computer system supporting AmbuQual for easy tracking and fast, permanent retrieval.

In Fremont, a specific form is used every time an indicator is formally reviewed. This simple, one-page form is called a "Monitoring and Evaluation Worksheet" (Exhibit 6), and it allows the organization to document exactly what is being assessed, by aspect and related indicator; the precise criteria and standards being used to evaluate performance; the data source and sampling methodology used; and the exact processes for monitoring and evaluation. When assessment yields a specific problem, a separate "Problem Identification Worksheet" (Exhibit 7) is completed, noting the specific problem, the action needed, who should take this action, and actual problem-solving

results (including specific improvements noted). This form
also documents the final date on which the problem was officially considered resolved, to provide historical tracking
information.

At MIT, a "Q.A. Review Form" (Exhibit 8) for defined
indicators provides documentation of the specific criteria addressed, results of the evaluation, and corrective action (both
recommended and actually taken). This form ultimately serves
as both a data source (reflecting a specific case audit and its
results) and a generator of corrective action. It also serves, in
combination with other documentation avenues such as memos,
reports to affected committees, and meeting minutes, to effectively track the noted problem to completion.

All of the programs we visited actively utilize perhaps the
most common of all documentation tools—meeting minutes.
This is, in fact, a perfectly acceptable way of tracking and
documenting identified problems and corrective actions as long
as the trail of decisions and actions is clear, the minutes are
complete, and the record is both permanent and easily retriev-
able. In order to help integrate Quality Assurance information
throughout the organization, minutes should also be appropriately distributed; at a minimum, copies should be sent to all
persons responsible for specific action, to the organization's
clinical and administrative management, and (as desired) to the
governing body.

Minutes need not be lengthy to be complete; often one or
two pages will suffice. At a minimum, the following four items
should be specifically documented:

1. *The convening of the meeting itself.* This shows that the neces-
    sary group process actually occurred. Specific note should
    be made of the date and who attended.
2. *The agenda addressed.* Identify the important aspects of care
    that were addressed, as well as the related indicators that
    were specifically monitored and evaluated.
3. *The decisions made.* In general, there are four possibilities
    here:
    a. All was well, and no further action was necessary.

Exhibit 5. AmbuQual Practitioner Performance Audit.

COMMUNITY HEALTH NETWORK, INC.
AND
METHODIST HOSPITAL OF INDIANA, INC.
PRACTITIONER PERFORMANCE AUDIT

Center _____ Chart #_____ Date of Index Visit _____

Practitioner _____ Auditor _____

INDEX VISIT

General Care   YES   NO   NA

1. Was the subjective data adequate?

2. Was the objective data adequate?

3. Was the assessment adequate?

4. Were the diagnostic procedures adequate?

5. Was the treatment adequate?

6. Was a consultation requested when indicated?

7. Was the follow-up interval appropriate?

8. Was patient education for acute and chronic problems adequate?

Continuity of Care

9. Was the patient given a return appointment?

10. Was the return appointment or referral for consultation tracked when indicated?

Cost-Containment

11. Were all diagnostic tests necessary?

12. Were all medications necessary?

13. Were all referrals for consultation necessary?

14. Were generic medications used when appropriate?

GENERAL CHART REVIEW

Continuity of Care

15. Has patient care been provided without significant interruptions in the treatment plan?

Exhibit 5. AmbuQual Practitioner Performance Audit, Cont'd.

INDEX VISIT

1. Documentation of the essential subjective protocol elements or reasonably sufficient subjective data to support the diagnosis, establish the prognosis or influence the treatment.
2. Documentation of the essential objective protocol elements or reasonably sufficient objective data to support the diagnosis, establish the prognosis or influence the treatment.
3. Documentation of an assessment which accurately reflects the subjective and objective data and includes the status of chronic problems.
4. Documentation of the essential diagnostic protocol elements or reasonably sufficient diagnostic procedures to support the diagnosis, establish the prognosis or influence the treatment.
5. Documentation of the essential treatment protocol elements or reasonably appropriate, safe and efficacious therapeutic plan including medication, dose and duration of treatment.
6. Documentation of the essential referral protocol elements or reasonably advisable consultation for diagnosis or treatment including the following:
   Treatment appears ineffective
   Diagnosis remains in doubt
   Worsening condition
7. Documentation of the essential follow-up protocol elements or a reasonably suitable follow-up interval.
8. Documentation of the essential patient education protocol elements or reasonably sufficient patient education related to the diagnosis, treatment and prognosis.
9. Documentation of a return appointment unless one has already been given or the patient receives primary care elsewhere.
10. Documentation of tracking for a return appointment when reasonably advisable or for any of the following:
    Incomplete immunizations
    Unresolved chronic problems requiring medications
    Scoliosis in children
    Abnormal Pap Smear
    Documentation of tracking for referrals when reasonably advisable.
11. The diagnostic tests were reasonably needed to support the diagnosis, establish the prognosis or influence the treatment and were not duplicated.
12. Medications were reasonably needed for effective treatment and were not duplicated. Medications were not significantly more costly than other medications which would be just as effective.
13. Referrals for consultation were reasonably needed for diagnosis or treatment.
14. Generic medications were prescribed when available and therapeutically equivalent to the innovator drugs with the following exceptions:
    Anti-psychotics or loop diuretics.
    Medications for patients > age 75 years with multiple problems or on multiple drugs.
    Medications for patients with problems that may be difficult to establish such as depression, asthma, diabetes, congestive heart failure or severe hypertension.
    Dilantin or Lanoxin.

GENERAL CHART REVIEW

15. Diagnostic tests and treatments which have been planned have been accomplished with reasonable continuity with the following exceptions:
    Patient has failed to adhere to the treatment plan.
    The plans have been appropriately changed.

**Exhibit 6. Washington Outpatient Surgery Center
Monitoring and Evaluation Worksheet.**

Department/Service: _____ Medical Staff _____ Date: ____ 11-6 ____

Major Clinical Function/Aspect of Care:

_____ Patient preparation for surgery or

_____ diagnostic/therapeutic procedure.

Indicator:

_____ Presence of informed consent.

Criteria:

_____ Written documentation of informed consent on Center

_____ chart. Less than 10% deficiency is acceptable.

Sample:

_____ 60 randomly selected patient charts.

_____ 20% of charts are deficient.

Methodology:

_____ Physician members of Quality Assurance committee

_____ review pre-op History and Physicals for documentation.

_____ Results compiled, Quality Assurance Committee, Board

_____ of Directors, and Medical Staff notified.

Data Sources:

_____ Dictated Pre-op History and Physicals,

_____ Center "Short Form" History and Physical.

**Exhibit 7. Washington Outpatient Surgery Center
Problem Identification Worksheet.**

Department/Service: _____ Medical Staff _____ Date: ___ 11-6-___

Identified Problem:

     20% of Pre-op History and Physicals have no

     informed consent.

Action Taken to Resolve Problem:

     1) "Informed Consent Given" section added to Center's

     History and Physical form. 2) Memo sent to Medical

     staff regarding necessity for documentation of

     consent. 3) Restudy of problem at next Q.A. (Feb.)

     meeting.

Responsible Person(s) to Monitor Resolution:

     Gerald G. Pousho M.D./Medical Director.

Assessment of Actions and Documentation of Improvement:

     February 26, 19__ Quality Assurance meeting – Review of 75

     charts (November, December 19__ and January 19__) 25%

     without informed consent. Plan – renew physician awareness,

     effort via memos to individual physician and medical staff.

     Restudy at May Quality Assurance meeting.

Date Problem Resolved:

     June 19

*Please include a copy of this worksheet in your department's report to the
Hospital Quality Assurance Committee.

Exhibit 8. Sample MIT Review Form.

Q.A. REVIEW FORM—ABNORMAL PAP SMEARS

PATIENT NAME _____ MR NUMBER _____

DATE OF TEST _____

REVIEWER _____ DATE OF REVIEW _____ INITIALS _____

Indicators of Appropriate Care	Present	Absent	Comments
1. Pap smear—*atypical, with koilocytosis.* Patient contacted within one week after report was received, advised to have repeat Pap smear in 4–6 months.			
2. Pap smear—*dysplasia, suspicious for malignancy or positive for malignancy.* Patient contacted within one week after report was received, advised to have repeat Pap smear and/or visit to Gynecology Service.			
3. Pap smear report was initialed by responsible provider.			

PROBLEMS IDENTIFIED:

ACTION RECOMMENDED:

ACTION TAKEN:

---

     b. Not enough data were available to determine whether or not a problem truly existed. (In this case, the Quality Assurance committee would want to go on record as calling for the needed additional data.)

     c. A problem (clearly specified) was identified.

     d. A potential problem was noted, and a special follow-up study was commissioned to ascertain the true scope or cause of the problem.

  4. *Problem tracking accomplished.* "Active" problems need to be continually reviewed, to ascertain their progress toward

resolution. And, as noted, problems that have previously been resolved should also be reviewed periodically, to ensure that they remain resolved.

Another frequent technique to initiate and track problem-solving activity is the common memo. Again, this is used to varying degrees in virtually every program we surveyed; in one program, memos in combination with some basic reports and meeting minutes constituted virtually the entire documentation system. The memo's advantages are that it is personal, informal, and capable of quickly generating or documenting action. It can, however, be *too* informal, and it may be more easily overlooked by the recipient than a more formalized message. In order to be most effective, memos should be officially documented in meeting minutes (as directing a specific action or reporting on action taken), and they should be routinely followed up (through stated deadlines, suspense files, subsequent notes or phone calls, and so on). Additionally, memos that represent direction provided on behalf of the Quality Assurance committee should probably be sent by, or over the signature of, the Quality Assurance committee chairperson.

Of course, each of the five studied programs deals with tracking and documentation in its own way, each with a differing degree of formality and each within its own specific context. For instance, at The University of Chicago Hospitals, Quality Assurance information flows upward through several hierarchical levels within a relatively complex structure; appropriate formal documentation must accompany each successive move of information (upward or downward).

In Indianapolis, as we have seen, there is a highly structured system of formal documentation and follow-up; the results find their way into a centralized program notebook, in which are kept the ongoing status of Program Quality Index and other scores, a current QIP log, agendas and minutes of Quality Assurance committee meetings, and so forth.

In Atlanta, while the ongoing business of routine assessment is handled somewhat less formally than in the other programs, Quality Assurance staff members are continually devel-

oping more formal instruments as part of the active transition to
a more centralized program.

Sample Documentation Systems. Because they involve excellent
views of total systems (formal, informal, and combined) that
result in effective documentation of problem solving, we will
track a specific "real-life" problem from each of two different
sites as examples of effective mechanisms by which problem
solving can be facilitated through appropriate documentation
techniques.

At the Washington Outpatient Surgery Center, one of the
specified indicators within the medical function deals with
ensuring documentation of informed consent actions in the
medical record. As shown on the Monitoring and Evaluation
Worksheet (Exhibit 6), the criterion for this indicator states,
"Written documentation of informed consent [will be] on center
chart." The specified standard for the criterion is 90 percent;
that is, as noted on the form, "less than 10 percent deficiency is
acceptable." In the course of evaluating organizational performance through a randomly selected representative sample of
history and physical documents, the reviewers (physician members of the Quality Assurance committee) noted that the sample
did not meet the stated standard. Therefore, as noted on the
worksheet, the results of the audit were distributed throughout
the committee, to the board of directors (representing the
owners of the center), and to the full medical staff.

Because a problem had been specifically noted, the committee also completed a Problem Identification Worksheet (Exhibit 7), also for appropriate distribution. The problem was
specified as "20 percent of pre-op history and physicals have no
informed consent." Clearly, this could be a potentially significant quality issue, with obvious legal implications. Therefore,
the committee worked through appropriate staff members to
ensure that history and physical forms specifically noted obtaining informed consent from all patients; in addition, a memo was
also sent to the medical staff underscoring the need for vigilance in this important area. Finally, the committee noted that
the problem would be investigated again at the next quarterly

meeting. The medical director (also serving as Quality Assurance committee chairperson) was named as the responsible party for corrective action.

Follow-up evaluation at the next committee meeting indicated that the problem had not yet been resolved. Therefore (as noted in the "assessment of actions and documentation of improvement" section of this worksheet), the committee made a new plan based on the distribution of individual memos to all physicians, as well as on creation of an article for the medical staff newsletter stressing the issue. Also, the committee again noted its intent to reevaluate the status of the problem at the following meeting.

At the subsequent ("May") committee meeting, seventy-five randomly selected charts were once again reviewed. This time, only two charts showed a lack of informed consent, and the committee judged the problem to be resolved. However, since informed consent is an ongoing indicator, the committee continually reviews the issue, even though the specific problem has been resolved.

Throughout the entire process, appropriate documentation was developed, and all involved parties were kept up to date regarding the status of the problem. A specific "log for tracking quality assurance activities" is kept current by the medical director for all identified deficiencies; this manual form provides ongoing details of problem description, date initiated, problem analysis, responsible person, stage of study, corrective action, follow-up, and resolution. This log, a simple block form that scans from left to right over two sheets of paper, is kept in a looseleaf binder to enable easy reference and updating on the status of all problems being tracked.

At each Quality Assurance committee meeting in which the problem of informed consent was discussed, minutes recorded the ongoing discussions and any resulting actions taken. In addition, subsequent minutes from meetings of the full board documented reports made by the Quality Assurance committee to the board on the issue of informed consent compliance.

The MIT Medical Department is, of course, much larger and more complex than the program in Fremont; one of the resulting dynamics is that ambulatory care is only one of many organizational components of the department (as shown in the organization chart found in Chapter Three). Such complexity necessitates even more compulsive documentation if tracking efforts are to be truly successful.

The problem we will follow through this system deals with abnormal Pap smears. This represents a situation in which all cases of "critical incidents" (here, Pap smears for which specific follow-up is called for) are reviewed and evaluated. The Quality Assurance review form (Exhibit 8) shows the criteria for care, by category of the specific abnormality. As with most of the criteria in use at this site, there is no specific standard noted on the form because there is effectively an implied 100 percent standard. Thus, all variances are reported to the Quality Assurance committee for further evaluation. When a problem in performance, as documented on the review form, is noted in any given case of abnormal Pap results, a formal memo is sent to the provider documenting both the finding and the action that needs to be taken.

At a regular meeting of the medical records committee, a formal report to the committee (made by the Quality Assurance coordinator) identifies the specific Pap smear problems in detail, as well as the corrective actions taken (memos sent, procedures changed, and so on). In addition, a review of previously reported cases explains prior problem resolution and reports specific case rechecks; this provides a valuable tool for continual tracking of prior problems. The meeting of the medical records committee routinely results in detailed minutes, which serve as an ongoing historical record.

The medical records committee, like all other committees and services that feed directly into the Quality Assurance process (see Chapter Three), makes formal reports to the Quality Assurance committee at least twice each year. Part of this report is a summary, on behalf of the ambulatory care services, of the ongoing Pap smear audit results. These reports are accepted (with suggestions and recommendations, as appropriate), and the results are duly noted in the formal monthly minutes of the Quality Assurance committee. The Quality Assurance committee chairperson then reports up the organizational line, first to the executive committee of the medical staff (to which the Quality Assurance committee directly reports), then to the medical management board of MIT. Throughout this process, a manual log of all variant cases is kept (in this instance, problems in follow-up of abnormal Paps); this log tracks the designated categories of Problem Identification Mechanism, Problems Identified, Action Taken, and Follow-Up. For each service or committee that feeds into the Quality Assurance process, a separate and detailed notebook of all issues relating to that group is kept, and one of the items routinely included is the ongoing log.

Reporting Activities

The needs for reporting are fairly straightforward. Quality Assurance should be reported through all appropriate channels as established by the organization; that is, each organization must decide for itself who should get what. There are, however, some commonly accepted "givens." Clearly the governing body needs periodic reports on the activities of the Quality Assurance program; it is also important to include the professional staff, as well as the chief executive officer (CEO) and perhaps all management staff. Finally, it is often useful to design the reporting system so that the entire staff is routinely made aware of Quality Assurance activities and issues.

Reporting can generally be handled by simply sending copies of the tracking documents, important memos, meeting minutes, and so forth through normal, preestablished reporting channels. The scope of reporting is a major continuing consideration; the documentation that is distributed must clearly note, within the constraints of appropriate confidentiality, the following issues:

1. Precisely what was discussed at meetings;
2. Specific decisions that were made;
3. Problems that were identified;
4. Who was requested to solve each identified problem; and

5.   The Quality Assurance committee's judgment concerning
     the potential significance of any given deficiency.

     Equally important is the frequency of reporting. Here, as
with so many other functions, there is no "right" time frame for
reporting. Each organization must again decide for itself how
often formal reports on Quality Assurance will be needed for
which receiving groups, depending on the size of the organization, the volume of patients treated, the number of aspects and
related indicators, the respective levels of the various groups
receiving the reports—the list of factors goes on and on. Within
our five programs, reporting intervals vary considerably, from
the daily Quality Assurance reports and entries made into the
staff communication book in Fremont, to the quarterly reporting to the board that occurs in the Atlanta and Chicago programs. The point is that virtually any reporting interval is frequent enough if it meets the real needs of the total organization
and provides the Quality Assurance function the continuing
visibility and credibility it requires.
     The reporting format also needs to be tailored to the
specific organization. Any number of avenues can be followed.
In Fremont, for example, the board receives a graphic Quality
Assurance trend sheet that quickly shows, through illustrative
trend arrows and percentages, the movement and magnitude of
performance changes for all specified indicators since the prior
report. At HealthNet, we use a monthly numerical index and an
accompanying line chart to show month-by-month progress.
Other programs simply use routine narrative reports and meeting minutes to get their points across to the organization. Again,
whatever works for the organization is what should be
employed.

Annual Program Review

     An accreditation requirement of the Joint Commission,
and a notion that makes a great deal of practical sense on its
face, is an annual appraisal of the Quality Assurance program
itself. It is obvious that in a field as dynamic—and as critical—as

Quality Assurance in the ambulatory care setting, both the overall discipline and the organization itself could experience significant change in a year's time; therefore, an annual look at whether or not the Quality Assurance process is serving the organization to best advantage is essential. Then, too, continuing positive debate regarding the Quality Assurance system and its attendant methods and results can only help stimulate thinking that will ultimately ensure that Quality Assurance remains a central theme within the organization.

All five of our study programs carry out such an annual program review, some informally, some through specified questions. (In addition, those programs that involve a number of organizational units or levels generally also encourage each to perform its own annual program review.)

In Cambridge, Bruce Biller asks three basic questions of the overall program (through the Quality Assurance committee):

- Is the Quality Assurance plan current and accurate?
- Should the program focus on anything new or different in the coming year?
- Do the year's results show any significant positive differences in performance or quality? If not, *why* not?

Biller also uses the annual review to assess the specific indicators being employed by the program and to replace or add to the existing ones, as needed.

At HealthNet, we ask ourselves (also through the Quality Assurance committee) the following specific questions, as defined in the AmbuQual users' guide entitled *AmbuQual: An Ambulatory Quality Assurance and Quality Management System.*

- How can we become better at evaluating the quality of care delivered within the HealthNet centers?
- What are we not monitoring that we should be?
- What are we actively monitoring that may be a waste of time?
- How can we improve the real day-to-day impact of the Quality Assurance program?

- How can the findings of Quality Assurance be more appropriately applied?
- How can we better relate our continuing education and in-service offerings to specific Quality Assurance findings?
- How can we more effectively evaluate the true cost of the care we deliver?
- What should be our major Quality Assurance emphasis during the coming year?
- How can we maximize total staff involvement in our program?

Following discussion and resulting recommendations for improvement by the Quality Assurance committee, the Health-Net managers' group meets to make final decisions regarding needed Quality Assurance program changes.

The University of Chicago Hospitals program also writes specific annual evaluation items into the Quality Assurance plan. As stated in this plan:

[The] annual procedure entails evaluating the Program in the following areas:
- Problem identification process
- Efficiency and productivity of the Quality Assurance Committee and the Clinical Operations Committee and Quality Assurance Department
- Effectiveness of the Quality Assurance Program's organization with respect to reporting lines, responsibilities, and authorities
- Monitoring of resolved patient care problems and improved patient care
- Identification of problems that are yet unresolved
- Department, Hospitals, and Medical Staff compliance with Quality Assurance Program.

Whatever the issues addressed or the methodology utilized, it is critical to review the Quality Assurance program and its results on a periodic basis. It is also productive to report the results of this evaluation through the same channels that exist for all other Quality Assurance reporting.

We have now completed our journey through the total "proven approach" (that is, the generic Quality Assurance model developed in Chapter Two). Conceptually, the model is rather simple; in practice, Quality Assurance program development, implementation, and integration can take literally years of hard work. As we have seen, quality is not something that can simply be "tacked on" to an existing organization; rather, it must be actively nurtured ("seeds and water") and continually promoted as part of the "corporate culture" until it actively becomes embedded in the essential fabric of the organization. Only when everyone in the organization fully integrates quality thinking into daily activity will optimal, long-term quality improvement become a reality.

PART THREE

ACHIEVING SUCCESS
NOW AND IN THE FUTURE

Chapter 12

Nine Essential Principles for Effective Quality Assurance Programs

There is much about the quality of care we do not, as yet, understand.
— Avedis Donabedian

"Quality" is hot, in the ambulatory care field as in the medical world generally. According to a *Hospitals* magazine article (Koska, 1988, p. 66), "What was once a chore is now a top priority, according to quality assurance managers." The proven model we have studied in detail throughout this book can help any ambulatory care organization effectively address this increasingly important area. If the logical steps for monitoring, evaluation, and problem solving that we have described are successfully followed, virtually any such organization will be able to take pride in a Quality Assurance program that enjoys real purpose, effectiveness, and "clout."

In this chapter we shall aggregate and summarize some of the most important underlying principles from our foregoing discussions. These nine principles are at the heart of the Quality Assurance process; if they are kept in the forefront during implementation or improvement of a Quality Assurance program, the result will be relative simplicity in program development, as well as real effectiveness in ultimate program design.

These concepts also address a number of "real-world" problems that new or developing programs often encounter and help to strengthen existing programs that may, for whatever reasons, be something less than originally intended. And as with our proven model itself, these principles apply to virtually any type of ambulatory care organization; they have been effectively employed in small centers, and in provider groups affiliated with large tertiary care hospitals. In short, they are both basic and generic.

What follows, then, is really a collection of the essentials of the overall Quality Assurance process and of specific program development.

Quality Assurance Is a Two-Phase Process

There are two broad phases in a total Quality Assurance program, each with its own role and separate mechanisms: monitoring and evaluation, and problem resolution.

Monitoring and evaluation is, in effect, the basic mandate of the Quality Assurance committee. It is the overall activity through which the organization looks at the quality of its total program in a continuing, systematic way. The purpose of this mechanism is to uncover existing problems or to facilitate active pursuit of opportunities to improve quality; it also serves to confirm and document compliance with selected standards.

Monitoring and evaluation begins when the ambulatory care organization formally commits to assuring itself and its patients that the highest possible level of care is being rendered. The actual assessment process starts with an inventory of the scope of services (of all types) being provided. The entity then selects the most important aspects of care within the defined scope of services and further delineates specific indicators of quality within those aspects. It then chooses criteria and standards against which to measure organizational performance for the selected indicators, and continually evaluates performance by comparison with these criteria and standards.

At times during monitoring and evaluation, a previously undetected or currently unresolved quality related problem will spin out; when this occurs, the problem resolution phase is activated. This separate process involves clearly identifying the finding as a quality related problem, referring the problem to the appropriate clinical or administrative manager for action, and tracking the problem through to final resolution.

All of our five study sites utilize this two-stage process; through this mechanism the overall quality level of an organization will, in stairstep fashion, be improved over time.

The Quality Assurance Program
Must Have Organizational "Clout"

A Quality Assurance program will simply not work if the problems that it identifies are not taken seriously. Consequently, the program's success depends on efforts by the governing body, the administration, and the medical staff leadership to ensure that assessment effort has real support and clear top-down commitment.

In a free-standing ambulatory care facility or system, support for the program can come directly from the governing body, whether a community based board (as at HealthNet) or some form of ownership group (as at the Washington Outpatient Surgery Center). At HealthNet, for example, the community board has specifically commissioned the Quality Assurance program and receives regular reports concerning the program's progress and significant identified problems; in addition, all HealthNet employees are made aware that the board has invested Quality Assurance with significant power to improve the overall program. In Fremont, the Quality Assurance committee reports directly to the board (made up of owners of the center) on a quarterly basis, reviewing the total assessment program for these investors.

Ambulatory care centers that are part of a hospital Quality Assurance program may enjoy a built-in "clout factor." Problems that are not solved at the level of the ambulatory care program itself would be referred to successively higher levels within the hospital structure. Such is the case, for example, at The University of Chicago Hospitals: although it is expected that problems will generally be solved at the level of the specific clinics (with the assistance of the related clinical department and, in the case of ambulatory care, the ambulatory care Quality

Assurance subcommittee), any unresolved problems can move up successively to the Quality Assurance committee of the full medical staff, the executive committee of the medical staff, and the Quality Assurance oversight committee of the hospitals. Ultimately, a problem could be taken up to the full board of trustees for resolution if needed. In addition, the top levels of hospital management have explicitly made clear their strong support of the total Quality Assurance effort.

The point here is simply that without a clear demonstration of commitment and support from the highest levels of the organization, the Quality Assurance program will never be able to operate with real effectiveness.

The Quality Assurance Program Should Be Clinically Based, Comprehensive, and Structured

Clinically Based. High quality *clinical* care is, after all, the reason for the existence of the ambulatory care organization; therefore, the major emphasis of Quality Assurance must necessarily be on improvement in the quality of the overall clinical program (that is, on strengthening the program's positive impact on the health status of its patients).

Of course, administrative matters are clearly not inconsequential to the Quality Assurance effort. In every practice there are many organizational and managerial aspects that are vital to the proper delivery of high quality health care. Patient satisfaction (as affected by waiting time, staff courtesy, appointment systems, telephone triage protocols, and so forth) is one such area that has been repeatedly shown to have a significant impact on the ultimate result of the encounter. Likewise, relevant policies and procedures, the education and training of the professional and support staff, incentive and disciplinary systems, and countless other administrative variables will have an effect — in some cases profound — on the overall quality of patient care.

It is, however, easy to fall into the trap of reviewing primarily administrative or fiscal material. These data are often more accessible and more readily understandable than some clinical information. It may also seem easier to fix apparently clear-cut administrative difficulties than to tackle more complex clinical problems, many of which may have a more emotional content.

To keep a program in perspective, therefore, focus the total Quality Assurance effort on the "dimensions" of quality that accompany our working definition of quality proposed in Chapter Four: effectiveness, efficiency, accessibility, acceptability, and provider competence. If the activities you are monitoring in your Quality Assurance program do not substantially relate to one or more of these five dimensions, they may not, in fact, have been good candidates for Quality Assurance consideration in the first place. Always ask, "Does the issue being addressed have the potential to affect the health of the patient?" If the answer is yes, then you are without doubt addressing an appropriate activity.

All five of our selected organizations address clinical quality directly. While all address administrative issues also, these issues always relate clearly to the delivery of patient care. In some cases, such as in Fremont and Chicago, separate organizational units deal specifically with quality issues from an administrative perspective. In others, monitoring of management issues that legitimately affect patient care is integrated into a single monitoring and evaluation approach. But none of these programs addresses any purely administrative issues that do not have a visible bearing on the quality of patient care.

Comprehensive. An overall Quality Assurance program should also be *comprehensive.* This simply means that the entire clinical program should be subject to active and continuing assessment through the monitoring and evaluation process. Clearly, clinical areas that are not actively assessed could contain problems that will be allowed to go undetected. Since undiagnosed problems are not likely to be solved, the organization's clinical care could be substandard even without the organization's knowledge.

This, of course, is why our Quality Assurance model includes an active identification of the total scope of services being delivered by an organization. Once this "inventory" has been defined, the Quality Assurance committee can then make sure that each important component is included in the overall assessment program.

The system in place at HealthNet serves as a good example of a comprehensive approach. As noted in Chapter Nine, the AmbuQual program moves from 10 broad parameters based on the organization's overall identified scope of care through 40 important aspects of care and ultimately to roughly 150 related indicators of quality. These indicators are both clinical and administrative, and they cover all of the important components of quality care as perceived by HealthNet.

Structured. Finally, the assessment process must be structured; a good synonym in this context would be "systematic." The Quality Assurance effort should be consciously designed to ensure total program review over a given period of time; this is often accomplished by the development of a prospective schedule of review activity. Some Quality Assurance committees use a "problem-of-the-month" approach, which generally involves no predetermined review schedule. This approach can sometimes be acceptable, since problems of current interest are being monitored; on the other hand, such an approach does not necessarily ensure that all relevant organizational activity will ultimately be reviewed.

Most of the five programs we surveyed have found it helpful to develop a prospective schedule of review activities. While the specific review periods differ, the very act of setting up a defined schedule of monitoring and evaluation in advance seems to have served these programs well. An excellent example is the program at Fremont, where the three separate components of the total Quality Assurance program—medical, nursing, and business—each have defined a full range of quality indicators to monitor routinely. Once each quarter, all indicators from each of these three components are summarized, reported to the Quality Assurance committee, and reviewed for further action. Thus, the Quality Assurance system as a whole essentially reviews the entire organization once every quarter.

The Quality Assurance Program Should Begin
at a Simple Level

There is no doubt that Quality Assurance can become very complex. However, many programs make the basic mistake of attempting to become too sophisticated too quickly — to run before learning to walk. Too often, these efforts are self-defeating. The result is a program that does not work as intended, with a consequent loss of organizational enthusiasm and support. A potentially meaningful process can easily lose its credibility through such an approach, causing Quality Assurance to become little more than a paperwork exercise with little real significance.

If, on the other hand, the principle of simplicity in initial design is employed, the basic mechanics of making Quality Assurance really work can be developed early. Begin by making the basic components of the two-phase Quality Assurance process as uncomplicated as possible. Since the entire assessment program, including the Quality Assurance plan itself, is designed to be reviewed and revised as needed each year, there will be plenty of opportunity to build more complex mechanisms into the program at a later date. In fact, the final generation of the system may not fully materialize until several review cycles have come and gone; there is really no need to try to build Rome in a day.

In illustrating this concept, JCAHO (Benson, Flanagan, Liffring Hill, and Townes, 1987, p. 11) cites an example of an ambulatory care program that was attempting to write treatment protocols as part of its initial Quality Assurance development process. As it happens, this was our own HealthNet organization. Since one of the conditions we see most commonly is diabetes mellitus, we decided (logically, we believed) that our first protocol should be written around this diagnosis. After several futile attempts roughly a year apart, we gave up and went on to significantly less complicated work. The reason: we simply did not yet truly understand the process of writing protocols, we were not yet fully comfortable with the mechanisms for gaining

provider consensus, and we had little idea how to make protocols actually work once written.

It took several false starts before we finally realized that we
were attempting to begin with one of the most complex of
ambulatory conditions. So we started all over again, but much
more simply. We wrote one protocol on acne, another on
pityriasis rosea, and yet another on pinworms. By doing this, we
got the mechanics of the process to work, and we were then able
to gradually take on protocols of increasing complexity. We got
back to diabetes only after seventy-four other protocols had
been developed.

If your Quality Assurance program is in trouble, we suggest you back off, perhaps even start over, make it *simple* to make
it *work*, and then build on that initial success and the resulting
knowledge gained.

The Quality Assurance Program Should Be Structured So That Problems Are Identified and Solved at Their Own Levels

All five of the programs we reviewed made this principle a
part of their Quality Assurance implementation in some fashion. Problems relating to quality of care should be actively
identified and resolved at the lowest possible level within the
organization. While this is not always easy, it is nonetheless
necessary.

A good example of the practical application of this principle can be seen in the Chicago program. Here, a well-defined
Quality Assurance structure progresses to the level of the board
of trustees of the entire hospitals system. Problem resolution,
however, is generally expected to take place at the actual clinic or
department level whenever possible; subsequent levels of the
Quality Assurance organization become involved primarily
when a solution is not forthcoming at these levels.

In Chapter Two we noted the concept of quality related
activities within the organization (quality control functions,
quality improvement activities, and the delivery of quality patient care). These activities should have their own built-in feed-

back loops; this reinforces the principle of action being taken at its own level.

The physicians, for instance, should already have functional systems in place to identify and solve their own problems. The best example is probably the peer review mechanism. In each of our study sites, this mechanism, although integrated into the overall Quality Assurance program, exists as a separate system on its own. (In the Atlanta program, this separate process even extends to "outside" physicians whose only contact with Southeastern Health Services is through contractual arrangements for provision of primary care in their own offices.) Within each peer review program, problems identified through the process are referred back to the provider in question, and this provider — not the Quality Assurance committee — is expected to solve the problem.

The same type of process should also be in place for nursing. Such, for example, is the case at the Washington Outpatient Surgery Center, where nursing as a major component of the total clinical program regularly addresses eighteen indicators of quality. While the Quality Assurance committee reviews performance regarding these indicators on an ongoing basis, nursing is expected to take first note of any developing problems and to undertake all possible actions to correct the problem before the Quality Assurance committee's review.

Other quality related systems should routinely be in place for lab, pharmacy, and radiology as well. In addition, patient satisfaction audits and other audit systems should already have their own feedback loops that will enable problem identification and solution independent of the formal Quality Assurance program.

Thus, the role of Quality Assurance is to ensure that problems are, in fact, being identified and solved at their own levels. If Quality Assurance determines that something has slipped through the cracks, then the overall Quality Assurance mechanism is activated to ensure that the problem is appropriately addressed. Utopia would be an organization in which the Quality Assurance committee had very little to do because, as intended, all quality related activities were functioning properly and all problems were being identified and solved independently of the formal Quality Assurance system.

The Quality Assurance Committee Does Not Actively Solve Problems

This principle is, of course, directly related to the preceding one. Although the ultimate objective of Quality Assurance is to resolve problems that affect patient care, this principle states that the Quality Assurance committee itself should not have the responsibility for actually solving problems. Every organization has a management structure (both administrative and clinical) whose function is to perform this task. The role of Quality Assurance is to evaluate the performance of the overall organization regarding issues that impact care and to identify those problems that are not being adequately addressed; Quality Assurance then refers these problems to the administrative/ clinical management of the organization for resolution. (Of course, the Quality Assurance mechanism also needs to track all identified problems, to ensure that they are permanently resolved.)

As we have noted elsewhere in this book, it is actually counterproductive to invest the power to solve problems in the Quality Assurance committee; such a course of action would signal the establishment of dual channels of problem-solving authority. Thus, while the Quality Assurance committee can (and should) make appropriate suggestions, and while the committee should be invested with the power to determine when a problem has been solved, the actual resolution of problems must ultimately come from the management structure of the organization.

This principle is actively applied at our study sites. It is, for example, stated explicitly in the Quality Assurance plan developed by the Atlanta program, and Frank Houser states that "problem-solving activities are handled by the specific departments; it is only by exception that the Quality Assurance committee assists in developing a solution."

The Ultimate Mission of Quality Assurance Is to Improve Human Performance

In a health care setting, quality (or the lack of it) occurs at the interface between human beings, between the patient and the provider or support staff. Problems that affect the quality of care generally occur for any of three reasons—inadequate or malfunctioning systems, a lack of required knowledge, or inadequate or inappropriate action. There are human beings at the end of any system; there are also human beings responding to any educational, training, or motivational activities. Thus, the task of improving quality will always be grounded in changing the performance of individuals.

It is therefore important that the Quality Assurance committee not allow itself to be automatically convinced that problems are necessarily resolved through obvious actions or system modifications. In fact, true problem resolution cannot be verified without constant reevaluation of the original problem.

An excellent example of the value of such periodic reevaluation in ensuring performance change involves documentation of informed consent at the program in Fremont (as described in Chapter Eleven). As you will recall, a routine chart audit revealed that 20 percent of the medical records did not contain specific informed consent; the organization's standard stated that no more than 10 percent of charts should fall into this category. As a result, the center's history and physical form was changed, and a memo was sent to the medical staff concerning the requirement for documentation of consent. Reevaluation several months later showed that the initial intervention had not had the desired effect, since 25 percent of the audited charts were still without the required consent; clearly, the performance of the providers had not yet been changed. Another, more intensive awareness-building campaign was undertaken, this time including individual memos to specific physicians. When charts were once again audited at the next quarterly review, the deficiency level had dropped to well below 10 percent; thus, the second intervention had, in fact, effectively changed performance.

The mission of Quality Assurance is not to generate memos or to introduce new procedures and systems or to develop special training programs; it is simply to facilitate appropriate changes in human (and by extension, organizational) performance.

The Quality Assurance Program Must Actively Involve the Provider Staff

Physicians, like anyone else, will respond most positively to any significant program change if they are actively involved in the design and implementation of that change. This is especially true when the program in question can easily be perceived as a threat to professional autonomy.

Sometimes, however, generating the necessary involvement of providers can seem like a Herculean task. Disinterest, active distrust of the process, or both can create significant roadblocks to the Quality Assurance program's best intentions. A few practical suggestions can help in overcoming this difficulty.

First, demonstrate the real value of the program. Quality Assurance clearly has the capacity to improve both the care rendered to patients and the status of the physicians within the program; it also has the power to actively help preserve professional freedom. If physicians truly buy in to these ideas, they will more readily view Quality Assurance as an opportunity rather than a threat. Conversely, if physicians state an active belief that Quality Assurance is not relevant to their daily practice, they should be strongly encouraged to specifically suggest ways by which to make assessment more functionally relevant.

Second, involve physicians in planning the Quality Assurance program. Extending physicians this courtesy and incentive will result in a much better-accepted program.

Third, do not diminish professional authority. The program must be structured in such a fashion that it does not, either in fact or in perception, limit the individual or group authority of the providers. The practice of medicine must clearly and visibly be left to the clinicians.

Fourth, encourage physicians to take the lead in developing system accountability. General public accountability is being increasingly demanded from the health care system, and providers must be shown that their own best interest demands that they be in the vanguard. They must clearly see that otherwise someone else outside of the organization may do it for them.

Fifth, use the system to publicly validate good care and excellence in performance.

Active provider participation can also be facilitated by organizationally placing the Quality Assurance committee itself under the medical staff, or by having a physician as chairperson. This is a common structural strategy, and one that is used in the majority of the five studied programs.

Substantial Investment Should Be Made in Initial Program Implementation

The program must be well structured from the very beginning, and substantial "up front" effort should be invested in making sure that the program is implemented properly. Three practical steps can give any new program a significant head start.

Education and Training. As with any innovation, a high priority must be given to staff education and training. Even a well-designed program will be jeopardized if insufficient attention is paid to ongoing education regarding Quality Assurance. The staff needs to fully understand the fundamental concepts of the monitoring, evaluation, and problem-solving processes; in addition, team members need to gain a feel for how the various quality related activities of the organization interrelate within the overall framework of the Quality Assurance program. And finally, staff members need to truly understand the role they all play in the continual improvement of quality throughout the organization. There are some excellent examples of useful training programs among our five selected study sites.

In Atlanta, annual continuing education offerings include a module on Quality Assurance that is made available to all staff members; in addition, all staff were initially given mandatory in-services on new standards related to patient satisfaction and the organizational code of conduct. At HealthNet, the Quality Assurance coordinator presents an annual in-service session on general Quality Assurance concepts and the specific AmbuQual system to each of the three health center staffs. In Chicago, the Quality Assurance department continually gives presentations on overall Quality Assurance, as well as on the specific hospitals' Quality Assurance program, to departments throughout the institution. At MIT, as we have described, new Quality Assurance committee members receive initial one-on-one training and are given materials describing the preceding year's activities. Then each new member is asked to develop one fresh indicator for his or her specific area.

Active Involvement of Staff. Whenever possible, the total staff (like the providers) should be involved in program development and implementation. Quality Assurance thinking must permeate the entire organization; all staff members should be actively invested in the Quality Assurance philosophy, as well as in the continuing functioning of the Quality Assurance program. In short, Quality Assurance must become an active priority for the whole staff.

One excellent idea is to write some degree of Quality Assurance activity into everyone's formal job description. Just this type of total program orientation has been developed at Southeastern Health Services. Each staff member was initially asked to help formalize his or her own job standards as part of the "Service Heralds Success" patient satisfaction program. These job standards then became part of a standardized, organizationwide "service package"; all staff members' job descriptions thus reflect their own specific quality related job standards, and employees are evaluated in part on these expectations.

Specification of Authority and Responsibility. Clear lines of authority and responsibility must be spelled out for all Quality Assurance activity, and these lines must be well conceived in the early development of the program. Both overall tasks and specific responsibility for various quality related activities that feed into Quality Assurance must be clearly defined.

Special attention should be given to detailing the authority of the Quality Assurance committee itself. The precise relationships of this committee to the administrative and clinical management structures of the organization should be made completely clear, and the relationship of both the committee and various management structures to the governing body must also be unmistakable.

Each of our five sites had paid close attention to spelling out these issues from the outset. The resulting structures ranged from the relatively straightforward system in Fremont to the much more complex structure in Chicago; regardless of type or complexity, however, each Quality Assurance program was completely clear about its relationships with the rest of the organization.

Summary

In this chapter, we have attempted to distill the essential principles underlying development of effective Quality Assurance. We have also integrated a number of practical suggestions which can help make virtually any assessment program truly work.

A final word is in order regarding the *cost* of performing first-rate Quality Assurance through the application of basic principles described in this chapter. It is absolutely clear that a program of the magnitude of Quality Assurance will not be cheap, in terms of both direct and indirect costs. Time is the basic commodity for Quality Assurance development and implementation, and this resource is generally neither inexpensive nor unlimited. But none of the five programs we surveyed had any real doubt that the payoff was worth the investment. As Houser said, "It's probably worth much more, and we'd be doing assessment even if we didn't have to." The perspective of everyone with whom we spoke was perhaps best summed up by Inge Winer, when she stated her "strong personal belief that Quality Assurance is inherently cost-effective, in terms of both financial and social costs."

Chapter 13

Responding to
Immediate Challenges

American medical care is undergoing its most drastic
upheaval since the dawn of the age of science. . . .
— Victor Cohn, "The Lost
Patient"

Throughout this book, we have viewed the workings of five
Quality Assurance programs in various ambulatory care settings. All of these programs are, to varying degrees, functionally
on the "cutting edge" of the field today; thus, we can look at them
and get a good feel for where Quality Assurance is today, as well
as where it seems to be heading for tomorrow.

In this chapter we shall draw upon the common experience of these and other programs to form some overall ideas
about what may occur soon. Along the way we shall address the
fundamental challenges currently facing ambulatory care Quality Assurance programs (as described in Chapter One), including what must be our ultimate challenge — the development of a
total Quality Assurance technology so powerful and sophisticated that it will enable us to actually *manage* quality routinely
within our organizations.

Ambulatory Care in the Near-Term Future

We recently convened a group of top managers, both
administrative and clinical, from the ambulatory care services
department at Methodist Hospital of Indiana (the 1,200-bed
teaching hospital that manages our own HealthNet centers). The

purpose was to generate ideas on likely directions for ambulatory care as an overall field in the 1990s, for our own internal planning processes.

Since this book deals with the development of Quality Assurance in the ambulatory care setting, we believe the resulting list of six major "predictions" can help put into context our subsequent discussion of the future of assessment in this arena. While we recognize that the following list represents the thinking of only one group of ambulatory care managers, we believe it will nevertheless serve to highlight some of the most important issues we will probably all face in the foreseeable future.

First, there will be substantial compensation changes for primary care physicians. These changes will increase the relative earnings of physicians in ambulatory care, and they will reflect both shifts in general medical economics and an increasing use of incentive systems for physicians (based on quality of care rendered, as well as on quantity of patients served). The resulting improvements in ambulatory care physician compensation will attract greater numbers of high quality providers to the field, as well as more physicians with a specific interest in assessment issues.

Second, "managed care" concepts (specifically involving ambulatory care physicians as "gatekeepers" of care) will continue to become more prominent throughout the entire health care field. This will force changes in the ambulatory care system as a whole. Specialists will become more closely tied to hospitals, as well as to the primary care physician "gatekeepers." Thus, the role of the primary care physician in the total health care system will become more significant. In addition, as managed care techniques become widespread, quality concerns will increasingly focus on issues of efficiency of care delivery and on appropriateness of care (including both overutilization and underutilization).

Third, communication technology will become critical. Computerized records, other computerized data, and the ability to instantaneously communicate (though computers) between the ambulatory care office and the hospital will have a major impact on practice patterns.

Fourth, ambulatory reimbursement mechanisms will change significantly. Something on the order of diagnosis related groups (DRGs) will be developed for ambulatory care within the foreseeable future, based largely on the inpatient DRG system currently in place. Like the hospital system before it, ambulatory care will then have to structure itself to respond to these changing reimbursement forces.

Fifth, a national data set will be developed for ambulatory care. We will all contribute to, and measure our operations against, this data set.

And sixth, quality as an overall concept, and Quality Assurance as a specific process, will become more prominent. Competition based on price will be superseded by competition based on quality. Increasingly sophisticated Quality Assurance programs will be developed to measure quality in ways that are not currently used. These programs will be linked to the communication technology noted previously, and most likely to reimbursement mechanisms as well.

Quality Assurance in the Coming Decade

We need next to apply some visionary energy to our main subject, in order to see where Quality Assurance will find itself in the years to come. It is safe to predict that one day a Quality Assurance professional will pick up a yellowed copy of this book and shake his or her head at the rudimentary notions of the old-time "experts." But what will the Quality Assurance system of that future time look like?

There are actually two stages through which we must travel if we are to cover all of the relevant territory. First, we must attempt to predict the progress of Quality Assurance in the near-term future. Since Quality Assurance is now in its relative infancy, there will inevitably be some significant movement over the next decade as the field continues to become a recognized discipline and more effective generator of organizational change. We have arbitrarily chosen a horizon of ten years for our near-term look; while the specific changes we envision may occur before a full decade has passed, we believe that the field ten years hence will look much as we will describe.

But long-term changes, both in Quality Assurance and in the health care field overall, will not allow us to rest at that point. We foresee a time when Quality Assurance will be absolutely integral to routine decision-making processes in health care, both within provider organizations and by various public and private entities. Thus, we also need to look at the long-term future for ambulatory care Quality Assurance, to a time when Quality Assurance methods are an inseparable part of the on-going act of *managing* quality on a nationwide basis. This will be the subject of our next (and final) chapter.

The near-term future for Quality Assurance in the ambulatory care setting will be based on the foundations already being built. Thus, while we do not expect any cataclysmic methodological changes, we do expect a continuing refinement and sophistication of techniques as ambulatory care Quality Assurance is required to become increasingly more effective and efficient. The uses to which Quality Assurance information will be routinely applied will broaden internally within ambulatory care organizations and will gradually expand to encompass a range of external applications, to the benefit of the health care system as a whole. For these reasons, Quality Assurance will become increasingly well accepted for its own sake, and Quality Assurance information will become both more reliable and more relied upon. In short, we see the near term as evolutionary, not revolutionary.

Over the next ten years, we look for the most substantial progress to occur in five areas, which largely parallel the major challenges in Quality Assurance today (as outlined in Chapter One). These areas are: (1) an increasing acceptance of Quality Assurance by physicians; (2) a growing acceptance by health care organizations of the inherent value of Quality Assurance; (3) the emergence of a clear national leadership in the Quality Assurance arena; (4) an increasing sophistication in Quality Assurance technology; and (5) the ongoing development of true Quality Management capabilities.

Acceptance by Physicians. A decade from today, virtually all ambulatory care physicians will have accepted Quality Assurance as a valid and worthwhile process. These physicians will have developed a consensus that Quality Assurance can, if performed correctly, have a real and positive impact on the health of their patients. Ambulatory care physicians will thus be quite willing to invest the time and energy needed to make Quality Assurance programs really work to optimum capability.

Physicians will also increasingly look upon Quality Assurance as an appropriate vehicle to help preserve professional autonomy, to provide them with needed public accountability, and to continually validate the high quality of care they provide. Physicians will be actively leading the ambulatory care Quality Assurance bandwagon; it is not a coincidence that in most of the five highly functional systems we studied, the major program development energy came from physicians.

As part of this growing provider acceptance of Quality Assurance, "peer review" will cease to be an emotionally loaded concept, and physicians will increasingly accept the notion that measurement by one's peers (against criteria and standards that are largely self-developed) provides both a positive means for promoting professional autonomy and a real opportunity to improve patient care. Protocols will become more common, and serious misgivings about "cookbook medicine" will give way to a belief in the necessity—and value—of more standardized care modalities based on a better understanding of the real relationships between specific clinical processes and resulting health outcomes.

Acceptance by Organizations. In ten years, Quality Assurance will be pervasive throughout the health care system generally, specifically in the ambulatory care environment. All types of ambulatory care organizations will be actively involved in Quality Assurance on a continuing basis, partly because their providers will demand it. And, as important, ambulatory care organizations will not be doing Quality Assurance solely because they *have* to, but because they actively choose to. The benefits of Quality Assurance to all parties involved in the health care transaction will have become fully apparent, and they will for all practical purposes be universally understood and appreciated. What is more, the real costs of performing (and acting upon) Quality Assurance will be generally understood and widely accepted as a legitimate and necessary expense of doing business. As we have seen, this distinctly positive attitude is already a common theme among our five model program sites.

In the future, competitive pressures will force more ambulatory care organizations to develop well-designed and highly visible Quality Assurance programs. This will be largely due to the reality that health care purchasers, both individually and through large insuring groups, will include quality of care considerations in their selections of providers and health care delivery organizations. Marketing departments will make increasing use of quality of care factors (published for all to see) in selling their products in this highly competitive environment.

The "bottom line" is that ambulatory care organizations will gladly invest the JCAHO-recommended 1 percent—or more—of their total budgets in Quality Assurance activity, and they will strongly believe that they have made a wise investment in their future.

This increasing organizational willingness to commit real resources to assessment has already produced one highly promising sign—the development of a growing national pool of dedicated Quality Assurance professionals, staff members whose sole responsibility is to nurture an organization's Quality Assurance program. These professionals currently come from numerous backgrounds, from physicians and nurses to administratively oriented individuals. While there is as yet no standardized curriculum, one will most likely develop in the near-term future; thus, a decade hence there will be recognized academic programs producing degreed professionals in the Quality Assurance discipline. These professionals will become standard in ambulatory care organizations of all types.

Recognized National Leadership. Leadership in the overall Quality Assurance field will coalesce nationally over the next ten years. As noted, we believe that the Joint Commission on Accreditation of Healthcare Organizations will ultimately become the undisputed health care Quality Assurance leader; other national Quality Assurance bodies will follow the directions established by this organization.

Over the next decade, there will be significantly fewer changes in the broad philosophy of Quality Assurance than we have witnessed in recent years. This conceptual stabilization will enable ambulatory care centers to develop well-grounded Quality Assurance programs, based on a recognized and accepted national model, that will enjoy an increased potential to be optimally effective.

With the emergence of a recognized national Quality Assurance leader, we will see ambulatory care organizations become responsive to a growing body of specified national indicators and standards. Clinical quality indicators developed for specific use in the ambulatory care setting will become the framework for ambulatory care Quality Assurance activities nationwide. Ambulatory care organizations, regardless of whether or not they aspire to external accreditation, will adopt these national clinical indicators, and they will actively employ them in routine Quality Assurance and internal management.

Simultaneously with a crystallization of clear national leadership, the potential will emerge for formal networking between and among Quality Assurance programs around the country. The Joint Commission clearly intends to lead the way in this development. Many ambulatory care organizations will ultimately be a part of this broad-based, and most probably computerized, Quality Assurance network.

Improved Methodologies and Programs. We will see a dramatic maturing in Quality Assurance technology (and resulting programs) over the next decade. Without the historical constant of significant change in assessment philosophy, ambulatory care centers will have the opportunity to allow their Quality Assurance programs to fully mature. As they do, improved methods will make assessment more effective.

First, in the near-term future, Quality Assurance programs will become both more highly structured and more comprehensive. Ambulatory care organizations will perform more real monitoring and evaluation in selected clinical and administrative areas, and they will gradually increase the number of these monitored areas as levels of organizational confidence in, and sophistication of, Quality Assurance technologies increase. Ten years from now, we believe, virtually all ambulatory care organizations will have a comprehensive and well-structured monitoring and evaluation system in place.

Second, programs will over time focus their growing energies more visibly on clinical issues. During the next decade ambulatory care professionals will realize which specific indicators really do have the potential to positively affect the health of patients; these indicators will become increasingly prominent in Quality Assurance as a broad consensus regarding their ultimate value materializes.

Third, by the mid 1990s, there will also be a considerably greater number of real outcome indicators in ambulatory care. Additionally, there will be general agreement as to the progressive levels and practical definitions of "outcome indicators" of all types. However, many structure and process indicators will continue to be valid, due in part to the complexities and inherent difficulties in developing unquestioned outcome indicators in the ambulatory care setting. (Also, as we saw in Chapter Six, it is commonly agreed that outcome measurement by itself cannot give a true picture of total organizational quality.)

Fourth, in the next ten years, more efficient data generation systems will be developed. The high cost of Quality Assurance relates almost entirely to the cost of accumulating needed data, and successfully addressing this issue will come to be of major importance. Computers will be intensively utilized in an attempt to generate and analyze these data more efficiently. More emphasis will be placed on statistically significant yet cost-effective sampling methodologies, using standardized minimum sample sizes and commonly accepted statistical techniques. Perhaps surprisingly, a number of ambulatory care organizations today actually accumulate *more* data than are really needed to perform effective Quality Assurance, and this adds unnecessarily to the cost of an assessment program. In the near-term future, this overabundance of data will be pared down to manageable dimensions, and Quality Assurance programs will become increasingly "lean and mean." This increased efficiency in data collection will also play a major role in the growing acceptance of Quality Assurance by providers and health care delivery organizations alike.

Fifth, there is no doubt that in the future there will be considerably more computer supported Quality Assurance, in both the inpatient and ambulatory care environments, than exists at present. Computerized Quality Assurance programs today are often greatly limited by the lack of true clinical information that is made a part of existing computer information systems. However, as software systems in ambulatory care become more clinically oriented, and as medical records become increasingly integrated into computer data bases, a vast data bank tailor-made for Quality Assurance evaluation activity will emerge. Much of the chart review work being done manually today will be done primarily by computer.

With a constantly improving technology and the decreasing costs of computerization, ambulatory care organizations of all sizes will be able to afford at least some computer support. Quality Assurance is a major area in which great untapped potential exists for substantial progress through increased computerization. Even ten years from now we may be in only the initial stages of true computerized Quality Assurance in ambulatory care, and we will probably be just beginning to experience the incredible potentials of this technology (locally and regionally, as well as nationally).

Sixth, Quality Assurance programs of the future will routinely measure, quantify, and compare their levels of quality, both internally and through reference to national standards. The ability of a program to actually quantify quality (as provided by the AmbuQual system, for example), and to use that information to improve program management, will become increasingly accepted, utilized, and refined in the ambulatory care setting. The growing ability to genuinely measure quality in a fashion that produces a readily comparable and continually updated index number will mark a dramatic leap forward in ambulatory care Quality Assurance technology. This will begin to occur routinely over the course of the next decade, and it will effectively usher us into a new era.

Toward "Quality Management." At the end of our ten-year horizon, ambulatory care organizations will be poised on the verge of finally being able to routinely manage the quality of clinical care they provide to their patients. The ability to truly measure quality and related organizational trends, and to compare these on many fronts with commonly accepted internal and external norms, will provide an incredibly powerful tool for governing boards, managers, and medical directors. It will provide data that can be utilized to analyze in depth the strengths and weaknesses of an existing clinical program. This understanding will in turn make it possible to plan and implement appropriate interventions, then to monitor them for effectiveness; such interventions will be based on verifiable knowledge of relative levels of quality. In short, managers will finally be able to actually manipulate quality.

"Quality Assurance," then, will ultimately evolve into "Quality Management." To be sure, basic Quality Assurance techniques will remain in place, and Quality Assurance philosophies and methodologies will still be important. But they will ultimately be considered only a set of specific means to the real end of Quality Management rather than as ends in themselves.

Quality Management is, of course, what we all ultimately want to do. Today we are developing the basic systems and methods that will lead us to this capability. If we can learn to truly manage quality, we can finally maximize the potential of all patients to achieve their own highest levels of well-being. And that, after all, is the ultimate goal of any health care organization.

Chapter 14

Toward the Next Generation: The Future of Quality Assurance

> Was Quality something that you "just see" or might it be something more subtle than that, so that you wouldn't see it all immediately, but only after a long period of time?
>
> — Robert M. Pirsig, *Zen and the Art of Motorcycle Maintenance*

The picture we have just conjured up of Quality Assurance ten years hence shows substantial evolutionary change from today's system. However, even this relatively close horizon does not adequately indicate the place we believe Quality Assurance will occupy over the long term in our country's health care system. While we cannot predict with any real certainty *when* Quality Assurance will reach its full potential, we are confident in our view of what this long-range evolution will probably look like. In this chapter we shall attempt to part the haze of the more distant future and peer into what lies in store for ambulatory care Quality Assurance.

A True Statistical Base

In its long-range configuration, ambulatory care Quality Assurance will be statistically based. It will be significantly more data intensive than it is today, and these data will be managed largely through the computer systems to which we have alluded. These systems will be both internally organized around, and

218

externally linked to, a national data base, to facilitate simple and quick comparison of overall quality of care between and among various ambulatory care organizations.

As Chapter Thirteen pointed out, the important feature of this national data base will be a set of normative numbers (perhaps ultimately one number) that will serve as a summary "quality index" for ready reference. All local, regional, and national indices will be in the public domain, affording both providers and purchasers (public and private) ready access to a full range of necessary statistics. The indices themselves, as well as the various component numbers composing them, will be adjusted for the severity of the individual cases seen in any given practice. The assignment of such "acuity factors" is already being undertaken in the inpatient setting; its expansion to the outpatient environment is a virtual certainty. In addition, the overall quality index of any given organization will also be adjusted for other specific qualifying circumstances, such as the existence of residency programs, the relative age of the practice, and so forth.

As part of this movement toward greater statistical basing, peer review and other individual case reviews will be considered less as ends in themselves and more as integrated components of the overall organizational effort. The "law of large numbers" will increasingly form the basis for the comparative system in which the quality index concept will be grounded. Single cases will still be judged on their own merits, but they will increasingly be seen primarily as factors contributing to a broader statistical base against which to analyze trends.

The past few years have witnessed the beginnings of this statistical basing. We have recently seen several new systems spring into being that purport to give an organization the ability to approach measurement of quality through various types of statistical compilations or up-to-date clinical data bases. We have discussed one such tool, the AmbuQual system, in this book.

Of course, numbers alone cannot provide the final evaluation of quality. In emphasizing this critical point, one unidentified reviewer of our manuscript recalled the classic question,

"How many laughs does it take to make a funny party?" The parallel is clear and cogent. We fully agree with this reviewer that continual quality improvement within an organization necessarily depends upon (in addition to improved statistical methodologies) an appropriate mind-set and shared value system among the total staff. Thus, a "corporate culture" that continually underscores quality, when taken together with the resulting professional commitment to quality concepts that must permanently infuse the work of each staff member, is a necessary precondition for effective Quality Assurance of any sort.

We believe that quality indices of the future will contain a built-in numerical factor allowing for all appropriate subjective judgments, as well as objective evaluations. Nevertheless, the heart of future Quality Assurance technology will be the reduction of all of an organization's separate reviews and individual cases to either a set of numbers or a single index number, enabling appropriate internal and external comparison.

National Indicators and Standards

Going hand in hand with the concept of national quality index computations is the notion of nationally published and commonly accepted indicators and standards. There is little "hard" common agreement now about what should be monitored and what should be expected, but the idea of a national quality index presupposes some universal guidelines based on a common idea of what such an index number entails.

Therefore, the ambulatory care organization of the future will not have to reinvent the wheel; it will have ready access to indicators and standards already developed, negotiated, and adjusted on a national level. This will make the task of developing a Quality Assurance program significantly easier and enable the same universal yardsticks to be applied to all programs.

Standards will most likely always have to leave room for some error in an organization, at least for as long as these organizations are run by human beings. But national standards will eventually point toward the zero defects level as the truly relevant standard, especially for those organizations that will have performed Quality Assurance for long enough to approximate such a standard in practice. While we will undoubtedly never fully achieve the ideal of a truly problem-free environment, it is nevertheless an ultimate standard on which we can legitimately set our sights at some point in the future.

An Outcome Orientation

Quality Assurance programs today are essentially doing relatively little real outcome measurement. And, as we have seen, there will always be a place for indicators relating to structure and process. However, anything less than the ongoing control of outcomes effectively shortchanges the organization, its patients, and the health care system as a whole.

Our Quality Assurance program of the future will not encounter this worry, since routine outcome measurement will be the rule rather than the exception. While JCAHO points out that outcome measurement is not necessarily an indicator of quality, such measurement is, in fact, commonly perceived as a primary vehicle for "flagging" potential problem areas. In the future, there will be common acceptance of what outcome measurement really is, of the various levels and types of possible outcome determination, and of what constitutes appropriate standards for each.

The Joint Commission has already begun to set the stage for the future in this regard. This body has publicly announced its intention to use outcome measurement as one major factor in granting accreditation for hospitals. As noted in the *Group Practice Journal*, the "initiative to base the hospital accreditation process on clinical performance measures and outcomes will have far-reaching effects on both hospitals and physicians" (Honaker and Robbins, 1988, p. 11). It is thus eminently reasonable to assume that defined outcome measurement will eventually find its way to outpatient physicians and organizations in the future.

Common agreement regarding outcomes will eventually be based on the existence of empirical data generated by rigorous longitudinal studies. The result will be outcome oriented indicators and standards that will be genuinely valid and, therefore, usable at a national level; these will be continually refined through constantly updating study results showing the effect on health status of various interventions and quality levels. It will be universally recognized that the most meaningful level of outcome review flows from the ability to accurately measure current health status, as well as from an awareness of predictable, cause-and-effect changes in that status, either for a single patient or for a representative group of patients.

Concurrent Quality Assurance Activity

For all practical purposes, Quality Assurance today is a retrospective discipline. Data collection is generally "after the fact"; peer review, as one example, is sometimes conducted as long as several months after the case under study has been completed.

Even so, for Quality Assurance to be optimally effective, it must facilitate needed change as near in time as possible to the event being investigated. As Biller points out, the operative idea is "to keep water from continuing to flow under the same broken bridge."

Future practitioners will have access both to the necessary technology and to prevailing attitudes to enable largely concurrent Quality Assurance. As medical records are computerized, as specific standards (and protocols based on these standards) become universal, and as Quality Assurance methodology becomes truly statistical, it will become a relatively easy matter to keep track of organizational quality indices. This will be accomplished through routine, up to the minute computerized status updates for all indicators addressed by the organization. Thus, needed quality related information will be virtually instantaneous throughout the organization.

Even more intriguing is the likelihood that at some point in the future, technology will allow immediate computerized quality checks for specific cases, through reference to universally accessible protocols and standards. An existing system, the Diagnosis Assessment Program developed by Massachusetts

General Hospital, already affords physicians the opportunity to verify diagnoses through comparison with computerized symptomologies for more than 2,000 diseases. In addition, an *American Medical News* article reported on expert testimony at a Senate Finance Committee health subcommittee; this testimony suggested that "the federal government ought to spend about 200 times as much as it now does to help the MD's and their patients find out which treatments work best" (McIllrath, 1988, p. 1). Clearly a universal and immediately available list of "best" treatments could easily form the basis both for concurrent Quality Assurance activity and for continuous provider ratings based on adherence to these proven treatments.

The future obviously holds fascinating possibilities for the concept of "instant" quality verification. When such a system becomes universal, the notion of Quality Management will begin to reach its true potential.

Resulting Incentives and Sanctions

Flowing logically from the concepts of national standards and concurrent quality review is the notion that Quality Assurance will move out of the realm of solely internal management and into the broader world of external decision making. As quality indices become reality, it will clearly be quite possible for outside organizations, both public and private, to make important decisions through review of the quality of any given ambulatory care provider or center. These decisions will ultimately entail both incentives and sanctions.

Incentives may be either formal or de facto through the marketplace. In either case, the incentives carrying the most weight will probably be at least partly financial; in other words, the buyers of health care (individuals and groups) will make purchasing decisions based mainly on who provides the best care at the best prices. While grounded in a national data base for which participation may be virtually mandatory, this external decision-making model is nevertheless firmly rooted in the ideas of free enterprise and competition.

On the public side, as questions on improved access to

care for all citizens come to the fore, government at all levels will increasingly make use of publicly available quality indices to make many types of health care funding decisions. The Health Care Financing Administration already utilizes institutional mortality data regarding Medicare hospital admissions; this is a big step toward routine comparison and rating of hospitals on the basis of quality, for the purpose of allocating public resources. Parallel systems for ambulatory care will at some point surely follow.

In the private world, corporate buyers of health insurance will increasingly look at both quality and cost in deciding where to put their health care dollars. The UAW, for example, already requires contracted HMOs to continually document medical outcomes and health status of member enrollees.

In both cases, public and private, the failure of an organization either to document its quality or to optimize its quality of care (as shown in its quality index) will in the future lead inevitably to missed financial opportunities. The handwriting on the wall is perfectly legible, and it carries an unmistakable message for those who choose to see it.

Walter McClure has already posited a specific health care purchasing system grounded in these concepts. He calls this the "Buy Right" system: consumers can either "Buy Right" by shopping for a health care provider on the basis of quality and cost, or "Buy Wrong." Either way, in large measure the choice of consumers drives this system, and one has to believe that as health care costs continue spiraling upward, it will not be long before consumers take up the "Buy Right" chant in growing numbers. As McClure (1987) has stated, "Purchasers don't yet realize they have this power, and most providers don't realize they've lost it. But in fact the change *has* occurred, and it's interesting to watch them wake up. . . ."

At some time in the future, this awakening will have been completed; at that point, quality and cost will become *the* bread and butter issues for ambulatory care organizations. In fact, movement has already begun in this direction. The *Group Practice Journal* noted in an article on quality, "Compelled by rising costs, employees, consumer groups, labor unions, and special interest associations have formed a coalescence to demand their dollars buy the maximum care" (Honaker and Robbins, 1988, p. 10).

The converse of incentives is also ultimately a pocketbook issue; this is the concept of *sanctions* based on quality index numbers. Just as public agencies can decide to purchase from a high-quality, high-efficiency provider for such public programs as Medicare and Medicaid, so these same agencies could withhold payments or simply switch providers based on a "default threshold" grounded in a quality index.

To the extent that one believes external accreditation has meaning for the future, a quality index also looms large as a generator of sanctions based on withheld accreditation. To cite the most obvious example, if JCAHO is to become the preeminent Quality Assurance leader, it is certainly not unthinkable that this same organization will in the future refuse (or withdraw) accreditation based on an organization's quality index status. In fact, the Joint Commission already withholds accreditation if an organization's Quality Assurance program is not found to be effective. Since JCAHO-accredited organizations are often "deemed" to be in compliance with requirements for participation in publicly funded health care programs, it is clear what such a sanction could mean to a health care organization.

It is also quite possible that future medico-legal decisions and sanctions will be based in part on results of external Quality Assurance information review. If, for example, a malpractice charge filed against a provider or organization could be adjudicated partly through reference to a commonly accepted quality index, and if that provider's specific index could be proven to be continuously below the specified minimum legal standard, this demonstrable lack of quality could conceivably make that provider de facto liable.

One final concept is a logical consequence of the idea of sanctions based on quality index levels. This is that Quality Assurance programs will more than likely be combined organizationally with risk management departments in the future. Since both responses to financial sanctions and defenses

against legal actions are within the currently recognized purview of risk management, this is a highly plausible place for
Quality Assurance within an organization.

In fact, some Quality Assurance programs already fall
under risk management departments (most notably in the hospital setting). Other programs, however, have actually been sepa-
rated from risk management functions. We believe this is a
completely understandable stage through which an organization might move before ultimately reuniting these two related
disciplines. Since rigorous assessment has only relatively recently been viewed as a critical undertaking, it is understandable that Quality Assurance could become a separate structural
element while it establishes both its own methodologies and a
necessary organizational identity.

However, we believe that in the long term, any organization with both a Quality Assurance component and a separate
risk management function will ultimately combine the two.
Current indications are, for example, that the Joint Commission
is heading in the direction of placing increasing future emphasis on risk management as being integral to an overall Quality
Assurance effort.

Effecting a Cost-Quality Balance

The major dynamic within the health care arena today is
the tension between costs of care and the quality of that care.
This dynamic will continue to drive health care well into the
future.

It is a short leap from the predictions above to the notion
that the discipline now known as Quality Assurance (and to be
known in the future as Quality Management) will have a profound effect on this dynamic. We believe it will become increasingly clear that this cost-quality tension does not, in fact,
have to be a zero-sum game, in which a gain on one side is
balanced by a loss on the other. We believe, as do countless
others in the field, that cost and quality issues can not only
coexist peacefully but also actively reinforce one another.

Walter McClure's "Buy Right" system, for example, proposes this win-win scenario. In his framework, purchasing decisions drive the overall system, and these decisions are made on the basis of inextricably bound cost and quality considerations. McClure (1987) notes that in a system driven solely by questions of cost, "'Joe's Cheap HMO' will buy cheap doctors." However, if quality considerations, facilitated by public review of Quality Assurance results, are included in the decisions made by purchasers, such "cheap doctors" will soon be out of business simply because no one will purchase their services. All we need do to set this system in motion is to accurately *measure* quality, then cause purchasers to want to "Buy Right" based both on quality and on the related concept of efficiency (which views cost partly as a by-product of quality).

Thus, Quality Assurance can indeed have a profound impact on the cost-quality dynamic that will set the tone in health care for years to come. And since, as we noted early in this book, the ambulatory care field will play an increasingly important role in the health care of the future, it is clear that Quality Assurance in the ambulatory care setting will be a powerful force well into the twenty-first century.

Summary

In sum, Quality Assurance is most assuredly not a passing fad. As more and more providers, purchasers, and health care delivery organizations become aware of the power and the potentials in the effective performance of Quality Assurance, the ambulatory care field will see an increasing reliance on this growing technology. In the future, Quality Assurance methodologies and resulting quality indices will be refined, quantified, validated, and used nationally to make vital health care decisions as part of national health policy. This, in turn, will further enable Quality Assurance to become a major force in the internal decision-making processes of the ambulatory care organizations of the future.

When we have finally arrived at true Quality Management, and when we can effectively use its techniques to routinely improve the health of our patients, we will know that the long upward climb will have indeed been worthwhile.

Resource A

Selection and Descriptions of the Five Case Study Sites

Our initial goal in selection of five specific programs to serve as case study sites was threefold:

1. To represent various areas of the United States, in order to show the common applicability of basic concepts, regardless of geographic region;
2. To include major different ambulatory care entities, in order to note peculiarities that might be specific to organizational type; and
3. To demonstrate various methods and systems representing excellence in Quality Assurance development and implementation.

In order to meet the first test (geographical distribution), we chose ambulatory care organizations from the East Coast, the South, the West Coast, and the Midwest. We will confess to what may at first seem regional chauvinism, since we included *two* midwestern sites. Issues of regional pride aside, we did so primarily to include our own AmbuQual Quality Assurance program as an example; this program appears to be a unique and, by all external evidence, quite usable system that comes as close as anything we have yet seen to actually *quantifying* the notion of "quality."

Our second imperative was to select varying types of organizations that would represent the major players in the broad ambulatory care arena. We selected an ambulatory surgery center; a proprietary group practice; a community health center network; a comprehensive, integrated health system with major prepaid/HMO involvement; and a major university affiliated, hospital based health services complex. While some sites actually represent more than one category (the proprietary group practice, for example, also happens to generate the major share of its business through HMO activity), these overlaps caused no real problems in our analysis.

Finally, we insisted on organizations known both for their general program excellence and for the strength of their Quality Assurance mechanisms, since these organizations were to serve as examples for other developing programs. We began by compiling a lengthy list of potential candidates; next, we investigated all possibilities by matching these candidates against our organizational and geographic needs. We ultimately selected five of the most appropriate sites that, in addition to meeting these tests, were also recommended by knowledgeable outside parties (including JCAHO ambulatory care surveyors).

We believe we have chosen five sites that essentially "cover the waterfront" with respect to both geography and organizational type, and which are known for the excellence of their operations, specifically their Quality Assurance programming. The structures (both of the parent organizations and of the specific Quality Assurance programs) and some salient quality related characteristics of these five sites are described below. Actual assessment methodologies from each program are addressed in the main body of this book; in addition, specific organization charts regarding the assessment-related structures of each entity are shown in Figures 2 through 8 in Chapter Three.

Southeastern Health Services

Located in Atlanta, Southeastern Health Services (SHS) is a proprietary group model practice, 85 percent of whose business is prepaid activity through PruCare (the HMO operated by Prudential Insurance Company). Another 5 percent of the organization's business is through a new preferred provider organization (PPO) also operated by Prudential, and the remaining 10 percent is other business. The group's thirty-six physicians are employed by a professional corporation that has a contract with Prudential; partnership is available after two years' employment. The group has five locations around Atlanta, with at least one site in each quadrant of the city. Hospitalization is at one of several Atlanta hospitals. Roughly 200 persons are employed by the organization, which provides approximately 200,000 patient encounters annually.

The group is multispecialty; in addition to departments of family practice, internal medicine, pediatrics, and OB/GYN, there is also representation from the fields of allergy medicine, ENT, dermatology, and orthopedics, and one of the internists has credentials in oncology. Capitated referral arrangements are in place for surgery and all needed inpatient services.

The group has been in existence since 1981, when it was formed specifically to contract with PruCare. Quality Assurance was part of the organization's original thinking, generated in part by the desire to become "federally qualified" through the federal HMO Act (which requires an HMO option for employers having more than a defined number of employees); the act did not, however, require a highly structured Quality Assurance system, and it dealt largely with credentialing, peer review, and patient complaint issues.

An assessment structure has been formally in place since the organization's beginnings. The department of quality control was formed in 1982, and the Quality Assurance committee was initiated in 1983. Since that time, SHS has produced ongoing reviews, annual work plans, monthly committee meeting minutes, and documented quarterly reports to the board of directors.

In 1987, SHS began to actively refine its assessment system, in order to prepare itself for seeking JCAHO accreditation (which Prudential desired for several reasons, including a wish for new Medicare business). The group subsequently received full accreditation; since that time, it has continued its Quality Assurance development efforts, working on improving the various quality related committee structures, formalizing Quality Assurance documentation, developing stronger feedback and follow-up mechanisms, and strengthening its trend analysis techniques.

One of the major program refinements was patient satisfaction. As part of the sophistication of Quality Assurance, a new emphasis was placed on the concept of patients' perceptions of quality. A consulting firm from Indiana was brought in for an intensive patient satisfaction development program; the result was the "Service Heralds Success" program, which became the most important ongoing interface between the line employees and Quality Assurance. Employees were integrally involved with the development of this program, helping to write the performance standards for their own job categories.

In addition, the specific Quality Assurance staff, known as the quality control department, began to be strengthened; as a result, Quality Assurance and utilization review functions began to be centralized. The director of quality control now oversees seven persons who monitor outpatient/hospital/referral network assessment, overall utilization, and member services.

The Quality Assurance structure also includes the Quality Assurance committee, headed by the medical director. This entity is actually a mandated committee of the board of directors, and was recently expanded to include the subcommittees of utilization management, risk management, medical records, pharmacy and therapeutics, and service (patient satisfaction). The multidisciplinary Quality Assurance committee itself consists of both providers and support personnel.

The committee meets monthly to facilitate the overall Quality Assurance process and to deal with identified problems. It reports to the full board of directors quarterly. While the Quality Assurance committee itself can specifically assign problem resolution activity when necessary, it encourages routine problem solving at the lowest possible level and receives reports of such action. While there is no formal instrument for tracking problem resolution over time, the group intends to develop one.

As part of the transition to a more formalized system, SHS began to prospectively specify important aspects of care, as well as indicators for those aspects. In addition, an annual Quality Assurance monitoring calendar was developed to provide a prospective schedule for Quality Assurance review; this calendar specifies some indicators for monthly monitoring, some for annual or semiannual monitoring, and periodic reporting dates for each of the assigned indicators.

Peer review audits are performed at least twice per year (the overall goal is quarterly) within each department or service. If any given service has only one provider, external providers are used for audit purposes. Additionally, SHS contracts with a number of independent family practice physicians in various locations, and these providers are subject to peer review audit once each year. As with other functions, peer review is becoming more formal and is being integrated more directly into the overall Quality Assurance process. For peer assessment activity, prevailing community or national criteria are used for comparison wherever possible, as in the use of American College of Obstetrics and Gynecology standards for timeliness of Pap smear testing. However, SHS is moving toward prospectively setting in-house clinical criteria and standards, to be developed by the group's own physicians.

Administrative issues that affect clinical care are also monitored through the Quality Assurance process. In general, subjective discussion and trend monitoring are the foundations of assessment in this area, which includes patient satisfaction surveys flowing from the new "Service Heralds Success" program.

Overall, Southeastern Health Services is a good example of a relatively less formal system in distinct transition to a more formalized program. More rigorous documentation and tracking mechanisms are being developed, as are more specific and prospective indicators and associated standards of clinical performance. The overall Quality Assurance program appears to be strongly supported from the top and generally well received throughout the organization, even though there is occasional resentment of quality control's perceived function of "looking over the staff's shoulder."

Some visible clinical improvements, such as implementation of an organizational mandate to overread all X rays within a specified time, have resulted from the discovery of potential problems by the Quality Assurance process. The only clear drawbacks to ongoing Quality Assurance, according to Frank Houser, are "the physician time required and the overall cost of Quality Assurance activity—but we're definitely willing to absorb both."

The MIT Medical Department

Just off bustling Massachusetts Avenue in the middle of Cambridge is the Massachusetts Institute of Technology; part of this sprawling complex is the relatively new building housing the MIT Medical Department. The department is in reality a highly integrated health care system serving the needs of students, faculty, and support staff (plus dependents) from the entire MIT family. With roughly 27,000 people in its patient base, the department provides approximately 120,000 ambulatory care visits per year through the services of nearly 225 department employees (slightly less than half of whom are physicians).

One of the department's components is a full-service student health facility that serves approximately 10,000 MIT students. Much like the department's HMO (described below), the student health activity is also prepaid; however, for this component, the prepaid revenues are held by the university itself.

With the exception of the student health service, the single greatest contributor of patients to the department is the MIT Health Plan, an HMO for nonstudents. Arnold Weinberg, medical director and MIT Medical Department head, says, "It is the HMO that makes this place different from other university health services; it is also largely the HMO that makes physicians want to come here." And it is through the HMO that major equipment purchases for the department are made.

The department makes virtually all major medical services available to its patients, including a complete range of primary care, ancillary services, psychiatry, social work, dental services, dermatology, ophthalmology, and other care. Such subspecialties as neurology and podiatry are also available. A unique feature of the department, and one that makes it a truly integrated and comprehensive health system, is the presence of an eighteen-bed hospital in the same building. Although the organization has affiliations with other major area hospitals (such as Massachusetts General Hospital, Children's Hospital, and others), the department also maintains its own fully self-sufficient hospital in order to provide greater continuity and comprehensiveness of care for its patients. The hospital also enables the department to bring patients back from other hospitals sooner than would otherwise be possible. The hospital provides roughly 1,000 admissions annually.

The department is fully accredited by JCAHO. During the year prior to the Joint Commission survey, a special group called the Survey Preparation and Evaluation Committee (SPEC) was initiated by the Quality Assurance committee chairperson. This group, composed of eleven persons representing several clinical and administrative interests, was also meant to promote Quality Assurance among the staff and the new medical director/department head. Following the JCAHO survey, the SPEC group was continued for the purpose of responding to the Joint Commission's recommendations.

Organizationally, the MIT Medical Department is responsible to both a medical management board and the MIT Corporation. As noted previously, the medical director of the department is also the department head; in addition, this individual serves as chairperson for the executive committee of the medical staff of the department and is a member of the medical management board. The department's ambulatory service is responsible to the medical director (through an associate medical director), while the Quality Assurance committee is one of many subcommittees of the medical staff's executive committee. The Quality Assurance coordinator reports to the department's executive director; together, this coordinator and the chairperson of the Quality Assurance committee manage the committee's activities.

The Quality Assurance committee itself meets monthly to facilitate the Quality Assurance function for the entire department. Through a preestablished annual review schedule, each appropriate medical staff committee and each service (including ambulatory services) makes formal reports of findings to the Quality Assurance committee at least twice each year. The Quality Assurance committee chairperson ensures that all meeting minutes are sent to the medical director, executive director, and the medical management board; additionally, the chairperson makes Quality Assurance activity reports on a monthly basis to both the medical and administrative staffs. Also, the medical director makes Quality Assurance reports to both the executive committee of the medical staff and to the medical management board. In order to tie all of these complex pieces together and to underscore the top-level commitment of the department to Quality Assurance, the medical director/department head meets with the Quality Assurance committee chairperson and the Quality Assurance coordinator on a regular basis.

These various reporting mechanisms ensure a strong tracking system for problem resolution. Findings of potential or verified problems are also routinely restudied following resolution, and an annual wrap-up report summarizes the various findings, resolutions, and other accomplishments of the Quality Assurance program.

The key element to the success of the overall program, according to Bruce Biller, is that monitoring and evaluation activity, as well as development of indicators and criteria/standards, are performed at the local level and are kept as decentralized as possible. In Biller's view, it takes a major leap of faith — which has proven successful within the department — to allow the Quality Assurance committee to *stop* doing Quality Assurance. The role of the Quality Assurance committee in this system is to facilitate local action. Investment of all staff members in Quality Assurance activity, as well as accountability by all staff for their own actions and the resulting impact on care, are Biller's guiding principles.

Another key element is Biller's insistence, with the Quality Assurance committee's concurrence, on "zero errors" as the legitimate standard for organizational and personal performance. In fact, everyone with whom we spoke at MIT underscored the notion that the universe within which the department functions is unusual in the general excellence of its membership; both the department staff and the patients who use the department's services are considered uniquely informed and uncommonly aware. Morale within the department as a whole is also generally seen as unusually good. For all of these reasons, the Quality Assurance system can, its developers feel, realistically promote expectations that are also unusually high. The bottom line in the Quality Assurance process is Biller's informal definition of quality as "a condition of 0 percent outliers and the permanent correction of errors."

The practical effect of this combination of maximum decentralization and what amounts to a general "100 percent standard" is that each reporting service or committee is left to develop its own indicators and to operate its own Quality Assurance process, with the underlying caveat that no deficiency (or opportunity to improve) is to be left uninvestigated. There are few specific clinical protocols as such; the organization chooses instead to focus its primary energies toward ongoing monitoring activity to ensure that clinical care is adequate.

An additional imperative in this program is that whenever a variance *is* noted at the local level, it is addressed immediately (and reported later). The notion of concurrent action is important in this system; the idea is to keep an identified problem from recurring while waiting for the paperwork to be completed.

Overall, the program appears to be quite well accepted at all levels of the department. It is strongly supported by the medical director/department head, who feels that the Quality Assurance program and its results add to the already high esprit de corps evident within the institution. The program also enjoys the active participation of the executive director, who sees the program as an excellent way to keep in touch with the clinical aspects of the organization.

Biller himself perceives many benefits from this strong Quality Assurance program. First, he says, it visibly promotes real excellence. Through regular Quality Assurance monitoring, for instance, the film repeat rate for radiology has hovered around only .8 percent for some time; the average national repeat rate is many times higher. Biller also notes that Quality

Assurance minimizes risk, both to the patient and to any organization that exists within a litigious environment. Finally, he feels strongly that Quality Assurance results in less costly operation of the total organization in the long run. Clearly, one person's stamp—Biller's—is strongly evident in the overall Quality Assurance program at the MIT Medical Department, and the vital and basically stable program that has now been in place for some time due to his efforts seems to be quite effective and well accepted.

Biller is not oblivious to the effect that the desire for external accreditation had on the organization's initial acceptance of Quality Assurance; however, he believes that the organization has now moved to a mode in which Quality Assurance is being driven from within the organization itself, for the primary purpose of improving the quality of care. As he says, "Initially, some people were only reluctantly supportive of the active process which led us to JCAHO approval—but the accreditation party was great! And we've now basically gone on to doing Quality Assurance for its own sake."

The University of Chicago Hospitals

At the edge of the Windy City is The University of Chicago, whose campus is home to The University of Chicago Hospitals. Although the hospitals system was recently made an entity separate from the university, its medical staff members still maintain faculty appointments in the university's medical school. The medical center itself includes more than 500 inpatient beds and a medical staff of more than 500, most salaried and working full-time at the hospitals. Approximately 100 subspecialty areas work out of twenty-five separate clinics in the hospital buildings. More than 200,000 ambulatory care visits are made each year.

The hospitals are accredited by JCAHO; this process served as an important catalyst for Quality Assurance within the institution. Inge Winer, Quality Assurance manager, says, "Because of desired changes to the Quality Assurance process, top-level administration became more interested in assessment issues and further educated themselves and the total staff regarding Quality Assurance." As part of this intensified process, Joint Commission assessment training sessions were attended by the staff, external experts were brought in to speak on Quality Assurance issues, and an educational journal club was begun.

The Quality Assurance structure in place at the hospitals is, of necessity, perhaps the most complex of the five sites we studied. This results from the fact that the hospitals system is a major tertiary care center providing both inpatient and ambulatory services; thus, its Quality Assurance plan and staff relate to both inpatient and outpatient care. Such structural complexity may well be endemic to a large university system, especially when overlaid with the requirements of a large and highly integrated medical practice.

Ambulatory care Quality Assurance begins with the individual clinics, where the day-to-day work of multidisciplinary monitoring and evaluation takes place. Each clinic reports to its immediate clinical department (for example, pediatrics), which receives monitoring and evaluation reports, helps recommend and assign corrective action, and performs first-line tracking and follow-up of problems or opportunities to improve care. These departments hold monthly Quality Assurance meetings.

Various subcommittees of the medical staff Quality Assurance committee, such as surgical case review, transfusion, infection surveillance, medical records, and utilization review, support the clinical departments and perform primary monitoring and evaluation within broad functional areas. There are ten of these subcommittees; one is the ambulatory care Quality Assurance subcommittee. These various groups meet on a monthly or bimonthly basis.

Both the clinical departments and the medical staff Quality Assurance subcommittees report their findings and appropriate follow-up activities to the Quality Assurance committee of the medical staff, whose function is to generally oversee clinical Quality Assurance. This entity assists with clinical Quality Assurance problems that cannot be dealt with at departmental or subcommittee levels, and it facilitates resolution of issues that may involve several subcommittees or clinical departments. The Quality Assurance committee meets twice each month.

The upward line of authority and responsibility just described is used primarily for clinical Quality Assurance issues. In addition, there is a separate organizational line for administrative/operational assessment issues, using a basically parallel process. Thus, ancillary departments and administrative committees/subcommittees report to a subcommittee of the clinical operations committee (COC), which is at a corresponding organizational level with the Quality Assurance committee of the medical staff. Therefore, both clinical and operational Quality Assurance functions are addressed in equal fashion.

Quality Assurance issues that for whatever reasons cannot be successfully addressed at the levels described above are sent for consideration and action to the executive committee of the medical staff (for clinical matters), and to the senior management group (SMG) (for operational matters). If a quality of care issue still cannot be resolved or bridges the division between clinical and administrative issues, it is forwarded to a joint medical staff/management committee known as the Quality Assurance Oversight Committee.

This oversight committee, comprising the highest levels of both medical and administrative authority within the organization, meets frequently to address quality issues and to develop the overall Quality Assurance system by considering needed modifications and program improvements. It is this body that provides essential coordination and oversight for overall Quality Assurance within the hospitals structure. This committee reports periodically on Quality Assurance issues to the full board of trustees, through the committee on professional responsibility.

Thus, the total structure is intended both to encourage each successive level to perform its own Quality Assurance function and to provide for general oversight and problem resolution. The Quality Assurance program as a whole has been moving toward more defined and prospective activity in selection of specific aspects, indicators, and standards/criteria.

Facilitating all of this activity is a dedicated Quality Assurance department, whose personnel assist all organizational levels in making decisions regarding what and how to monitor, in collecting data, and even in facilitating the needed reviews. The department also serves to ensure needed tracking, follow-up, and documentation of Quality Assurance activity throughout the entire system.

The Quality Assurance department was originally a part of the department of medical-legal affairs for the hospitals. However, with the increasing emphasis on Quality Assurance as a specific activity, the department was made a separate unit. As of this writing, the Quality Assurance department is combined with the utilization review function; however, while these units together form one overall entity, they both have their own dedicated staffs.

One of the major challenges faced during initial development of the specific ambulatory care Quality Assurance program within the overall hospitals structure was the sheer number of organizational components and the resulting complexity of monitoring and reporting activity. This necessitated a Quality Assurance mechanism that, while able to deal with these complexities, would nevertheless be as integrated, simplified, and unified as possible.

These mandates led to the development of a standardized monitoring format (shown as Exhibit 2 in Chapter Nine). Each of the ambulatory care clinics utilizes this format to monitor its own area twice per year, on a prospectively scheduled basis, through a one-week "block sampling" of specific aspects and indicators. During a sampling week, each ambulatory care clinic performs a continual review of all specified high-volume or high-risk procedures (which essentially equate to aspects of care), and clinic personnel routinely note all respective complications (which are basically indicators of quality). In addition, the unit chooses two "clinic-specific criteria" that need not relate to the other selected procedures and aspects and need not necessarily be high-volume or high-risk; they need only be of stated importance to the clinic itself.

The choice of procedures and complications is left almost entirely to each individual clinic, with little prospective over-

242 Excellence in Ambulatory Care

sight of the selection. However, the total Quality Assurance program is moving toward generally broader indicators, as well as ledger-based standardized reporting (especially to the board of trustees).

The system is in transition to a more integrated, formalized, and standardized approach to Quality Assurance. This activity is also becoming more overtly outcome oriented, and program developers are attempting to make the system as concurrent as possible, to assure that problem resolution and quality improvement occur speedily. An especially exciting development has been the institution of computerization within the Quality Assurance function, through which specific corrective actions and their results can be tracked over time.

As noted, the system is moving away from solely diagnosis-specific indicators toward broader indicators. In addition, the Quality Assurance function is beginning to address risk management issues more specifically. As a result of such changes, new areas for monitoring have emerged; relatively recent additions include ongoing 100 percent review of selected procedures, regular evaluation of drug usage, and continual assessment of continuity of care.

According to Winer, there is an unspoken consensus (as at the MIT Medical Department, the other university-affiliated site) that a "100 percent standard" should prevail in ongoing evaluation. However, for relatively less critical clinical indicators, lesser standards may be based on acceptable national practice norms. Active development of specific site-selected standards is an objective for future program development.

The Quality Assurance function is, in general, well received and actively supported within the broader institution. While initially there was some physician and staff resistance to formalized assessment, the program has now evolved to the point at which it is generally quite well accepted. Says Winer, "Most University of Chicago Hospitals physicians are full-time academic physicians and are research oriented. Thus, the conceptual base behind Quality Assurance appeals to them. Our physicians don't hide their difficulties, but they may not always be *aware* of problems in clinical care. It's part of the Quality

Assurance function to coordinate communication and feedback on quality issues."

Certainly a factor in this general acceptance of Quality Assurance is external accreditation. However, according to Winer, the system has now moved to a point at which Quality Assurance is valued for its own sake. "We certainly like the outside approval," she remarks, "but we now want to create the tightest ship possible for our own reasons. And we especially want to focus on ambulatory care issues, since that seems to be the way of the future. My personal vision is that as a university, we will become an acknowledged leader in the conceptualization of Quality Assurance. We are striving to be recognized as an expert resource in this area."

Washington Outpatient Surgery Center

Fremont, California, is a mid-sized town in transition from a farming economy to a professional base. It essentially serves as a "bedroom community" to the San Francisco Bay Area. Since 1986, Fremont has been home to the Washington Outpatient Surgery Center (WOSC), a proprietary ambulatory surgery facility.

The center is a joint venture between a local public inpatient facility, 250-bed Washington Township Hospital, and forty private physicians. While the hospital is the leaseholder for the portion of the building occupied by the center, it is not officially represented on the WOSC Board of Directors; rather, the center's board is strictly physician based. Seven providers make up this board, which meets bimonthly.

The center is the smallest (as well as newest) of the five organizations we visited. There are twenty-five persons on staff, including five employees in the business office and twenty nursing/technical staff members. Roughly 3,000 patients are treated annually, and more than 4,000 procedures are performed; these include all minor surgeries, such as endoscopies, excisional biopsies, cataract removals, arthroscopies, and so forth, but no major invasive surgery.

Given the size and age of the center, as well as the highly

specialized nature of its function, one might anticipate that the Quality Assurance mechanism would be reasonably uncomplicated. Such is, in fact, the case; the Quality Assurance structure is relatively less complex than in most of the other sites, and the number of routine aspects and indicators is relatively small. Specific standards are at this point fairly broad; as Magda Cockerline noted, "Right now, we are basically laying down a big net over the whole program, and picking it up constantly to see what we might find. More detailed work on additional specific indicators and more explicit standards will most likely develop over time."

This absence of complexity, however, clearly does not indicate a lack of effectiveness. The Quality Assurance system developed at WOSC is actually a highly functional program based on shared staff values, a nurturing corporate culture, and the capacity for immediate feedback.

Reporting to the board of directors is a Quality Assurance committee, which meets once per quarter. This group includes the medical director (who also serves as the committee chairperson), the director of nursing, and four physicians of varying specialties. This group oversees the total Quality Assurance program, receives summary assessment reports from the rest of the organization, makes its own reports on Quality Assurance issues to the full board, performs both random-sample and case-specific chart audits, and directs corrective action as needed.

The real work of the Quality Assurance program, however, is at lower levels. There are actually three areas of functional Quality Assurance; each operates through its own separate organizational channel.

Nursing Quality Assurance is the responsibility of the director of nursing. Reporting to this position is a Quality Assurance nurse, who spends roughly twenty-four hours each month in data collection for the nursing Quality Assurance function.

Medical Quality Assurance is the responsibility of the medical director (an owner of the center). A major function of this position is daily review of the charts of all persons receiving surgery, both prospectively and retrospectively. This is accomplished through a checklist of such issues as verification of surgeon credentials and privileges, inspection of preoperative lab reports, and dictation of postoperative discharge summaries. In addition, the physician members of the Quality Assurance committee perform a quarterly chart audit; this involves assessment of randomly selected charts for such general items as indications for surgery, as well as case-specific review of all charts displaying such "critical events" as hospital admission subsequent to surgery.

Business office Quality Assurance primarily addresses functions accomplished by medical records personnel, such as specific procedural charting issues.

Much Quality Assurance activity for all three of these functions occurs on a daily basis. Specific data sheets and summary tracking forms are used to routinely document assessment activity within each function. In addition, a communications book with updated information on day-to-day Quality Assurance issues is available to all staff members, and the daily "morning report" addresses Quality Assurance items as needed. Thus, as a practical matter, Quality Assurance activity is largely concurrent; each function is strongly urged to take its own needed action immediately, whenever a quality related problem occurs (then to report on these actions later, as needed). To this extent, the program largely promotes a decentralized evaluation system; the Quality Assurance committee actively intervenes in problem resolution only when lower-level action is for some reason insufficient.

Once each month, the entire nursing and business office staffs meet together to conduct general business. One of the major agenda items for this meeting is the presentation of specific Quality Assurance information, including a routine summary report extracted from the ongoing Quality Assurance logs. These monthly reports are then aggregated quarterly and presented to the full Quality Assurance committee.

The stated purpose of the Quality Assurance program is to assure the best patient outcome, the most cost-effective care, overall patient/staff safety, and an environment acceptable to both staff and patients. Specific aspects of care and related indicators of quality have been defined within each of the three functional areas (nursing, medical, and business office); the Quality Assurance committee reviews summaries for all aspects and indicators each quarter. The committee notes trends and assigns follow-up actions. Specific problems are documented on a special problem identification worksheet, which outlines the problem itself and tracks all corrective action to the point of final resolution. All problems are restudied at a future time, to ensure that they are fully resolved and that no recurrences are experienced.

A good example of this overall process can be taken from the nursing area. Written policy identifies six specific aspects of care: qualifications of the staff, physical facilities, equipment and supplies, documentation of care, documentation of significant variances in care, and cost-effectiveness. Flowing from these aspects are eighteen specific indicators of quality, including such items as infections, complications, hospital admissions, and statcrit controls (a quality control function). Each indicator is assigned a standard, with "zero problems" the underlying (if unstated) objective for each. For instance, under the indicator "charting deficits," the specific standard reads, "Less than 1 percent entry errors per month is acceptable *if corrected*" (emphasis added by the authors). An ongoing Quality Assurance log is kept for each indicator; as noted, a summary report for each is presented quarterly to the Quality Assurance committee, which discusses specific indicators as needed. In addition, a Quality Assurance trend sheet is prepared to facilitate review of the full set of nursing indicators; this sheet tracks ongoing improvements in the status of each indicator over time.

Two hallmarks of this Quality Assurance program are immediacy of feedback and day-to-day involvement of the entire staff, facilitated by the size of the organization and the general simplicity of the Quality Assurance structure and process. These factors also help explain the relative ease with which the Quality Assurance program was initiated, as well as the general lack of staff and provider resistance to assessment. In reality, the Quality Assurance program and the center itself began almost simultaneously; additionally, the staff has been essentially hand picked, in part for general attitude toward the Quality Assurance process.

The result is both an evident "family" feel at WOSC and a truly cooperative spirit regarding the need for assessment. This makes the job of assuring quality through a formalized process less taxing than is sometimes the case. While the organization has taken great pains to become fully accredited, Quality Assurance appears to be an idea whose inherent value is generally well accepted. As Cockerline states, "We all pretty much buy into the idea that working in a setting such as ours without a strong Quality Assurance component is like trying to dig a hole with a rake. Quality Assurance is absolutely integral to what we do for a living."

According to Cockerline, the assessment function serves three primary purposes from the staff's perspective: It generates recognized improvements in the quality of patient care; it provides a channel for ongoing communication within the total organization; and it reduces staff stress by providing a mechanism through which physicians and employees can exercise a measure of control over their own environment. She also believes that the WOSC system can be replicated in similar organizations; in fact, several other ambulatory surgery facilities are adopting the WOSC system.

In sum, the Quality Assurance program is both effective and well received throughout the center. While stable, it is nevertheless actively evolving and developing increased refinement. Cockerline's only real concern echoes that of several other persons we interviewed—that Quality Assurance can take significant staff and provider time away from actual patient care.

Community Health Network, Inc.

HealthNet, as our own organization is most commonly known, is a system of three community health centers located in Indianapolis, Indiana, a city considered one of the rising stars of the Midwest. The centers are funded mainly by the federal government to provide primary health care to "medically underserved" (that is, largely indigent) populations. Nearly 40,000 physician visits are provided each year to about 12,000 patients.

Each center has ten to fifteen staff members (including physicians); in addition, there are roughly fifteen centralized administrative and program support positions, making a total of nearly sixty employees. The system includes eight full-time staff physicians in family practice, pediatrics, and internal medicine. Each facility is the responsibility of a registered nurse who serves as clinic manager, and each center houses both a clinical staff and business office personnel.

HealthNet is operated by a community-based board, with representation from each local community; the total system is contractually managed by Methodist Hospital of Indiana, a 1,200-bed tertiary care teaching hospital. The HealthNet centers specialize in whole-person care, utilizing a strong network of referral providers. HealthNet's service package, in addition to routine physician care for acute and chronic conditions, includes health education, social work, outreach, counseling, and perinatal care coordination.

HealthNet's Quality Assurance system (the mechanics of which are discussed further in Chapter Nine) is probably the most highly structured of the five programs researched for this book. Built around a specific and recurring monitoring and evaluation cycle, the overall system is contained in a user's manual that walks the Quality Assurance committee step-by-step through the entire process. All aspects of care and related indicators of quality are reviewed once each cycle, which takes from a year to a year and a half to complete. The program is comprehensive; within a full cycle, more than 150 individual indicators representing 40 specified aspects of care are assessed. These aspects and indicators are tied to broad "parameters of care" that address all major facets of care delivery.

The name given to this system is AmbuQual, short for "ambulatory quality." A critical feature of the system is that it results in a numerical value of quality for each indicator; when aggregated, the total of all of these values is a single number that serves as an ongoing index of the overall level of quality within the HealthNet program. Thus, we can take a "snapshot" of our organizational quality level at any given time, to tell us how we are doing relative to our performance a month ago, six months ago, or at the same time last year. Since AmbuQual also allows us to view the specific numerical values of any individual aspect or indicator, we can also use it to begin to address real quality management by identifying the long-term effects of program interventions.

AmbuQual also enables us to specifically tailor the system to desired levels of quality and resulting corrective effort. One key to this concept is that all criteria/standards are determined in advance of actual monitoring and evaluation work; that is, for every indicator, a desired "level of quality" is specifically assigned by the organization's directors. Problem resolution can then be undertaken when the score for any indicator falls below the assigned level. One spin-off of this is the ability to set priorities for quality related efforts; thus, if the organization feels that a certain indicator, while important, is less critical than others, that indicator can be assigned a relatively lower numerical limit for corrective action, thereby ensuring that efforts will not be expended quite so quickly on that issue.

Another key to the prioritization of quality related effort is the Quality Assurance committee's mandatory assignment of deadlines for corrective action. Thus, if a problem is identified within a less critical indicator, the deadline for problem resolution can be set relatively far into the future.

Accompanying the detailed process for routine assessment is a highly formalized documentation/tracking system. A specific form called a quality improvement plan (QIP) is used to explicitly document any identified problem. This form describes the problem in detail, assigns a specific person to resolve it, sets the deadline by which resolution must be completed, and (by signature and date) documents the resolution.

All of AmbuQual's varied reporting and documenting processes can be performed manually; in addition, the system readily lends itself to computerization. We are now at a point within HealthNet where virtually all major tracking and reporting mechanisms are computerized.

While the process of assessment through AmbuQual is

highly refined, the organizational structure of the Quality Assurance program itself is basically quite simple. A multidisciplinary Quality Assurance committee is empowered by the community board to oversee the total assessment program. This committee answers to the executive director of HealthNet, and it makes formal reports to this person, the community board, and the Quality Assurance structure at Methodist Hospital. In addition, a dedicated Quality Assurance coordinator has responsibility for continuing program development and refinement of AmbuQual.

AmbuQual spells out quite specifically the role of the Quality Assurance committee. In short, the committee's job is to evaluate all aspects and indicators via a predeveloped schedule, to report on all problems discovered, to assign necessary corrective action, and to track problems and corrective actions to final resolution. A cardinal rule is that the committee does not solve problems itself; it may, however, make constructive recommendations. In addition, the committee may also send formal "memos of concern" to appropriate managers regarding evaluations that, although not below the specified QIP levels (standards), nonetheless involve issues for which improvement would benefit the organization.

The committee, whose membership rotates annually on a staggered schedule, includes representation from all functional categories within the HealthNet system: physicians, other types of providers, administrators, clinical support personnel, medical records secretaries, and so forth. We believe strongly that quality involves everyone in the organization, including the "troops in the trenches"; this fosters a balanced decision on every indicator, and it helps ensure that each relevant perspective is considered throughout the assessment process.

The AmbuQual system addresses all appropriate issues, both clinical and administrative, affecting the quality of care. One tough lesson we learned early was that administrative issues to be evaluated must have clear relevance to clinical quality in some way. In the early days of our Quality Assurance program development, the Quality Assurance committee produced numerous calls for problem resolution of a purely administrative nature; since a number of these were not clearly related to clinical quality, and since the sheer volume of these calls for action inundated the administrative managers (occasionally affecting the managers' ability to set their own priorities), the result was some early resentment of Quality Assurance.

Since the development of AmbuQual, however, this resentment has virtually disappeared. In its current form, our Quality Assurance system is generally quite well accepted within the organization, partly because it actively involves virtually all managers in a positive way, and partly because it has demonstrated a real ability to identify and help solve some difficult problems. (Even so, we must note that the Quality Assurance committee chairperson recently received a short memo that in its entirety read: "If you allow any more QIP's to be assigned to me, I'll break both your legs!" We have so far presumed that the note was sent in jest.)

In sum, we believe that AmbuQual successfully helps us quantify the organizational level of quality, and thus helps us approach the ability to actually manage quality within HealthNet.

Resource B

Sample
Scope of Services
Reviews

This Resource includes samples of how three of the study sites developed an initial scope of services review (Step Two in the generic Quality Assurance model outlined in Chapter Two). While the same general information is addressed by all three programs, each also has its own unique approach based partly on the structure and purpose of the organization. The real significance of these examples is, of course, that the respective organizations have made a conscious effort to specifically define what they do.

　　1. *Southeastern Health Services*, a full-service group practice working primarily with HMO/managed care patients, details the range of physician services and the related ancillary services it provides (including nutrition and health education). It also specifies the various staff categories providing these services, as well as hospital and specialty referral arrangements. (See Exhibit 9.)

　　2. *The University of Chicago Hospitals* is a complex organization with many types and levels of functions and disciplines within a large teaching and research environment. There is a specific Quality Assurance plan for the ambulatory clinic structure; this plan includes the "scope of care" (Exhibit 10). This description addresses both the general types of ambulatory care services provided and the major specialty/subspecialty clinics themselves.

　　3. *The Washington Outpatient Surgery Center* is strictly a

provider of ambulatory surgery services. Therefore, its scope of services review is essentially a six-page inventory (of which one page is displayed in Exhibit 11), by specialty, of all specific procedures performed at the center.

Each of these scope of service reviews is primarily clinical. In addition, as noted in Chapter Six, it is also useful to address organizational/administrative functions that directly enable the provision of high quality clinical care; these functions should also be monitored by the Quality Assurance program. For example, within our own HealthNet system, the review of care-related services that eventually generated our specific aspects of care included administrative policies (such as confidentiality and waiting time), general procedures (such as medical records and patient scheduling), environmental and safety programs, job descriptions (addressing such items as required education and experience), and so on.

Exhibit 9. Southeastern Health Services, Inc.: Scope of Services.

Southeastern Health Services, Inc., is a multispecialty group practice providing comprehensive medical services in the following specialties:

Internal Medicine, including	Ancillary services provided:
Hematology	Audiology
Nephrology	Chemotherapy
Oncology	Endoscopy
Family Practice	Health Education
Pediatrics, including	Lab and X-ray
Pediatric Immunology and	Nutrition
Rheumatology	
Ob/Gyn, including	
Certified Nurse Midwifery	
Subspecialties:	
Allergy	
Dermatology	
Orthopedics	
Otolaryngology	

Professional staff at SHS include physicians, physician assistants, nurse
practitioners, certified nurse midwives, registered and licensed practical
nurses, registered dieticians and accredited record technicians. Services are
provided at five office locations in metro Atlanta. We are affiliated with four
area hospitals and a referral network of over 150 specialists.

Source: Southeastern Health Services, Inc. Reprinted by permission.

**Exhibit 10. The University of Chicago Hospitals:
Ambulatory Care Quality Assurance Plan (Extract).**

Scope of Care:

Outpatient diagnosis, treatment and follow-up care is provided by all clinical
specialties and most subspecialties including Dentistry, Oral Surgery, Medicine, Surgery, Pediatrics, Ophthalmology, Neurology, Ob/Gyn, Radiology,
Radiation Oncology, and Psychiatry. Primary and specialty care is provided
including the following: primary care, secondary care, and health maintenance for adults and children; normal and high-risk obstetrical care; ambulatory surgery; follow-up care for inpatients; diagnosis and management of
chronic illnesses such as asthma, diabetes, cardiac problems. There are
approximately 250,000 visits per year to the ambulatory clinics.

Source: The University of Chicago Hospitals. Reprinted by permission.

Exhibit 11. Washington Outpatient Surgery Center:
Scope of Services (Extract).

General

Condyloma excision
Cyst excision
Debridement
Fistulectomy
Foreign body excision with/without
    X-ray
Ganglionectomy
Gynecomastia excision
Hematoma drainage
Hemorrhoidectomy
Herniorrhaphy, adult, pediatric, in-
    guinal, umbilical, ventral
Incision and drainage
Lesion excision
Pilonidal cystectomy

Pleurocentesis
Rectal polypectomy
Rectal dilatation
Sigmoidoscopy
Skin grafts
Suture removal
Thoracentesis
Torticollis repair
Tumor excision
Sinus tract excision
Varicose vein ligation with/without
    stripping
Varicocelectomy wound closure,
    secondary

Urology

Circumcision
Hydrocelectomy
Meatotomy
Orchiectomy
Orchiopexy
Penile condylomata excision
Penile pros. insertion
Prostate biopsy
Spermatic vein ligation
Spermatocele ligation
Testicular biopsy
Undescended testes repair

Vasectomy
Vasovasotomy
Varicocelectomy
Cystoscopy
Retrograde pyelography
Urethral dilatation
Internal urethrotomy
Cystometric studies
Scrotal exploration
Stone manipulation
Transurethral resection bladder
    tumor

GYN

Bartholin cystectomy and
    marsupialization
Cervical polypectomy
Cervical cerclage
Cervical biopsy

Hymenotomy/ectomy
Hysteroscope
IUD removal
Laparoscopy, diagnostic

Source: Washington Outpatient Surgery Center. Reprinted by
permission.

Resource C

Selected Aspects and Indicators

This Resource displays samples (in the originating formats) of selected "aspects of care" from three of the study programs, as well as some "indicators of quality" chosen for their relationship to these aspects. (Each sample comprises roughly one page of respective aspect/indicator listings which are substantially longer.)

    1. *The MIT Medical Department* has developed a chart detailing all important functions to be regularly reviewed (essentially a listing of aspects of care), with specified indicators to be included for each (see Exhibit 12).

    2. *Southeastern Health Services* combines its listing of aspects and related indicators with an annual calendar, arrayed by month, for prospective scheduling to review each item throughout the year. (See Exhibit 13. The calendar is not shown in the exhibit.)

    3. *Community Health Network* (our HealthNet centers) produces a manual on how to use our AmbuQual Quality Assurance program. One of the items in this manual is a detailed indicator inventory, grouping specified indicators under their "parent" aspects of care and assigning a scoring weight to each (see Exhibit 14).

Exhibit 12. The MIT Medical Department: Indicators of Quality.

Function (Aspect)	Indicators
Administration	Appointment backlogs Assignment of personal physicians Denials by Consultation Committee

Ambulatory Services	Quality of care, all clin. svcs.
	Mgt. of cases w/abnormal lab values
	  • Abnormal Pap smears
	  • Abnormal thyroid function tests
	  • (etc.)
	Abnormal mammograms

Patient Advocacy	Patient complaints about admin. procedures, clinical care, billing
Radiology	Accuracy of radiol. interpretations Repeats of suboptimal films
Safety/Disaster Prep.	Environmental safety (building systems, equipment, etc.) Fire and disaster drills Incidents involving safety

Source: The MIT Medical Department. Reprinted by permission.

Exhibit 13. Southeastern Health Services, Inc.: Indicators of Quality.

Clinical Quality (Aspect)

Specific screening criteria (Indicator)
- Admission for possible adverse results of outpatient management
- Abnormal test results/physical findings not addressed by physician
- (etc.)

Target diagnoses
- Asthma
- Drug Overdose (intentional)
- (etc.)

Department Reviews
- After-hours
- Family Practice
- (etc.)

Risk Management

Incident Reports
Fire and Code Drills

Pharmacy and Therapeutics

Errors

Administration

Appointment Availability
Credentialing
(etc.).

Source: Southeastern Health Services, Inc. Reprinted by permission.

Exhibit 14. Community Health Network, Inc.: Indicators of Care.

(Parameter of Care: "Provider Staff Performance")

Aspect of Care = Credentials
  *Indicator: Educational Background (1.0)
  *Indicator: Professional Experience (1.25)

Aspect of Care = Clinical Performance
  *Indicator: General Clinical Performance Audit (1.5)
  Indicator: Problem Focused Clinical Studies (.5)

(Parameter of Care: "Accessibility")

Aspect of Care = Ease/Timeliness of Access (Appointments)
  *Indicator: Appointment Triage System (.7)
  *Indicator: Appointment Procedures (.7)
  Indicator: New Patients — Routine (1.0)
  Indicator: New Patients — Acute (1.0)

(Parameter of Care: "The Medical Record System")

Aspect of Care = Clinical Information Availability
  *Indicator: Timeliness (.9)
  *Indicator: Content and Format (.9)

Aspect of Care = Provider Medical Record Documentation
  *Indicator: Problem List (1.5)
  *Indicator: Medical Record (1.3)
  Indicator: Family Profile Documentation (.6)

Note: * fundamental indicator — suggested for all organizations.
Source: Community Health Network, Inc. Reprinted by permission.

Resource D

Glossary

AAAHC. The Accreditation Association for Ambulatory Health Care. Like the Joint Commission on Accreditation of Healthcare Organizations, or JCAHO (in which AAAHC was originally based), this national organization surveys and accredits health care organizations; unlike JCAHO, however, it concentrates its efforts solely on ambulatory care organizations. Quality Assurance system review is part of its survey process.

Acceptability. (See Dimensions of quality)

Accessibility. (See Dimensions of quality)

Accreditation. Certification from an accrediting body (such as JCAHO, AAAHC, or NCQA) that an entity has met predetermined standards of organization and/or performance.

Ambulatory care. Health care provided to patients in settings other than inpatient hospital areas or the patient's home. The Joint Commission on Accreditation of Healthcare Organizations (JCAHO) lists the following examples of ambulatory settings:

> College or university health programs
> Community health centers
> Ambulatory care clinics
> Group practices
> Health maintenance organizations
> Independent ambulatory surgery centers
> Emergency care centers
> Urgent care centers

AmbuQual. A highly structured, computer assisted, quantitatively based system of ambulatory care Quality Assurance developed for use in primary care settings by Methodist Hospital of Indiana, Inc., and Community Health Network, Inc. (Indianapolis, Indiana).

Appropriate. Having a reasonable chance to positively affect the patient's health in a cost-effective manner. Appropriate care neither undertreats nor overtreats the patient.

Aspect of care. A significant quality related component of a health care program; it is one of many such components that flow from a "scope of services" inventory conducted by the organization. When taken with other aspects of care, it provides a functional evaluation of organizational performance.

Assessment. The process of comparing performance against selected criteria and standards. Basically equates to the "monitoring and evaluation" phase of the overall two-phase Quality Assurance process.

Audit. A structured system to continuously generate data needed for Quality Assurance monitoring and evaluation activity. It obtains information from a larger sample, generally through asking specific questions.

"Clout" factor. A necessary component of effective Quality Assurance activity that brings into play the commitment to performance assessment and problem solving of the highest levels of the organization (primarily the governing body and organizational management).

Criterion. A specific rule for decision making or performance evaluation.

Data. Information (either objective or subjective). Provide the necessary means to compare actual performance with a standard of perceived quality.

Data source. Where to find information needed to evaluate performance relative to established organizational standards for indicators of quality.

Dimensions of quality. Five primary facets of quality in health care, as first described by Heather Palmer (1983, pp. 14, 15). These dimensions, in Palmer's words, are:

> *Effectiveness.* The power of a particular procedure or treatment to improve health status.

Efficiency. The delivery of a maximum number of comparable units of health care for a given unit of health resources used.

Accessibility. The ease with which health care can be reached in the face of financial, organizational, cultural, and emotional barriers.

Acceptability. The degree to which health care satisfies patients.

Provider competence. [Concerned] with the provider's ability to use the best available knowledge and judgment to produce the health and satisfaction of the patient. . . [can] also refer to a health care delivery site and the way in which it functions as a whole.

Effectiveness. (See Dimensions of quality)

Efficiency. (See Dimensions of quality)

Empirical. Based in actual practice, as opposed to "normative."

Evaluation. Comparison of actual performance with pre-established criteria and standards. This comparison may be based on actual data or on subjective judgment.

Explicit. Objective and predetermined, as opposed to "implicit."

Functional. Performing or able to perform a specified activity; it works as planned.

Generic indicators chart. In the AmbuQual system, an all-inclusive list of parameters of care, associated aspects of care, and indicators of quality. Also included in the chart for each indicator are categories of information necessary for evaluation of that indicator, as follows:

Criterion
QIP level (Standard)
Data source
Weight
Scoring category ("Qualitative" or "Quantitative")
Responsibility focal point

Implicit. Subjective; based in opinion or judgment (often by "experts"), as opposed to "explicit."

Indicator of quality. What is actively monitored to determine how well the organization is doing with respect to a related aspect of care; an important subset of an aspect of care. Each indicator is important to monitor as part of an overall Quality Assurance program. Each should have its own standard, and each has the potential to affect the health of the patient in some fashion.

Indicator score. In the AmbuQual system, a number (0–100) awarded for each indicator. It may be "qualitative" or "quantitative" (that is, either subjectively or objectively assigned).

JCAHO. The oldest of the existing health care accrediting bodies (begun nearly forty years ago), the Joint Commission on Accreditation of Healthcare Organizations, or "Joint Commission," provides certification that organizations are meeting predetermined standards on structure and performance relating to quality health care. The Joint Commission has an overall ambulatory care division; subunits of this division specifically address managed care and ambulatory surgery. The Joint Commission focuses major attention on Quality Assurance as part of the accreditation process. Much energy is now being invested in developing outcome indicators that can become part of an ambulatory care organization's ongoing quality related effort.

Joint Commission. (See JCAHO)

Managed care. A system of providing care in which the "care managing" provider accepts responsibility for the total care delivered. Managed care implies an acceptance of financial and legal risks for full delivery of all appropriate care.

Management. The level in any health care organization at which primary activity is overseen and directed. Includes both clinical and administrative management.

Monitor. To review something on a continuing basis.

NCQA. The National Committee on Quality Assurance. Housed with, but separate from, the Group Health Association of America (the professional association for health maintenance organizations), this entity reviews and accredits HMOs and other prepaid health plans. Its primary focus is on Quality Assurance and medical records.

Normative. Based on a conscious decision regarding what "should be," as opposed to "empirical."

Outcome. The results of all related efforts to provide care. Can be of several different types and levels, as described in Chapter Six.

Parameter of care. In the AmbuQual system, a critical perspective of an ambulatory care program that, when included with all other parameters of care, provides a complete picture of the quality of the program. AmbuQual lists ten such parameters (as described in Chapter Nine).

Patient satisfaction audit. An audit system for obtaining information from a sample of an organization's patient population regarding satisfaction with the organization, the care received from it, and resulting health status.

Peer review. The process by which the performance of an individual provider is evaluated relative to a reasonable expectation of care. The review is carried out by another practitioner of the same discipline (often, although not always, of the same specialty); thus, physicians review physicians, dentists review dentists, nurses review nurses, and so forth.

Performance audit. A "peer review" audit of the performance of an organization's providers, based upon the medical record. Generally collects information that only a member of the provider staff is competent to evaluate.

Problem resolution. The second phase of the two-phase Quality Assurance process. When the first phase ("monitoring and evaluation") identifies a problem (or opportunity to improve), this phase ensures that the identified problem is solved (or the opportunity to improve is taken advantage of).

Problem solving. The act of accomplishing the "problem resolution" phase of Quality Assurance.

Procedure audit. An audit of the medical record to assess how well procedures are performed and documented by provider and support staff. It is often designed to be performed by clerical personnel.

Process. Specific activities involved in providing or enabling the provision of care (standard support staff procedures, accomplishment of specific protocols, and so on).

Program Quality Index (PQI). In the AmbuQual system, a quantitative summation of the quality of an ambulatory care program. It is derived from the average score of the ten parameters of care times their respective weights.

Protocol. The foundation for an explicit peer review process. The protocol defines a reasonable expectation of care. Protocols frequently, although not always, include diagnostic and treatment criteria, as well as documentation criteria. The criteria in the protocol should be predetermined, clinically valid, and developed by the professional staff who will be participating in the peer review process.

Provider competence. (See Dimensions of quality)

Provider staff. Those persons who, as a primary part of their jobs, make independent judgments that can directly affect the patient's health.

QIP level. AmbuQual term equivalent to "standard" (and roughly equivalent to "threshold"). The QIP level is the score below which management intervention becomes mandatory. A quality improvement plan (QIP) is generated by the Quality Assurance committee whenever the score for an indicator is below the QIP level. The QIP level is set by management and can be revised at any time.

Qualitative indicator. Indicator in the AmbuQual system for which a score is derived from a subjective judgment by Quality Assurance committee members regarding fulfillment of the related standard and the probable impact of any deficiencies on patient care.

Qualitative score. An AmbuQual score between 0 and 100, obtained by converting a subjective judgment made by the Quality Assurance committee regarding performance level into a numerical score.

Quality Assurance. A structured and comprehensive system to monitor and evaluate the entire clinical care program and to resolve deficiencies in that care when discovered.

Quality Assurance committee. The group (generally multidisciplinary) that functions as the organizational focal point for monitoring/evaluation and resulting problem resolution.

Quality control. The process of preventing unwanted or negative change.

Quality (in health care). (From the Institute of Medicine, 1974, p. 1): Care that is "effective in bettering the health status and satisfaction of a population, within the resources that society and individuals have chosen to spend for that care."

Quality improvement. The process of facilitating desired or positive change.

Quality improvement plan (QIP). In the AmbuQual system, a form for defining, tracking, and documenting resolution of problems identified in the monitoring and evaluation phase of quality assurance.

Quality patient care. The clinical result of combining effective quality control and quality improvement activities.

Quantitative indicator. Indicators in the AmbuQual system for which there are objective data that can be compared numerically against the preestablished standard for the indicator.

Quantitative score. An objective AmbuQual score obtained from data compiled by management or from results of audits (a number between 0 and 100).

Scope of services review. The process by which an organization essentially defines itself and its services (of all types). The resulting "inventory" of services facilitates selection of specific aspects of care to be monitored and evaluated. Scope of services review is also required for JCAHO accreditation.

Standard. A numerical marker (or model) of acceptable performance for any given criterion. Can be generated locally or based on national models.

Structure. The necessary resources that enable provision of care (method of organization, staffing ratios, policies, job descriptions, and so forth).

Support staff. Those staff members in an ambulatory care organization whose job is to support the provider staff in some manner in the care of patients. Includes medical assistants, receptionists, cashiers, lab techs, and X-ray techs. Nurses and therapists may be classified as either provider staff or support staff, depending upon their role in a particular organization. (See also Provider staff)

Threshold. A term developed by the Joint Commission on Accreditation of Healthcare Organizations (JCAHO) to prospectively describe how close an organization must come to meeting a criterion before in-depth, second-level evaluation must be initiated.

Training. Supervised experience for learning skills. This may be the clinical part of an educational program or an in-service offering by an employer.

Trend. A pattern of occurrence or performance, as noted over a period of time.

Two-phase process. The sum of the two major components of the generic concept of Quality Assurance. These two phases of Quality Assurance responsibility and activity are:

> monitoring and evaluation
> problem resolution

Weight. In the AmbuQual system, an explicit indication of potential impact on the health of the patient. For purposes of scoring quality levels, AmbuQual assigns weights to parameters of care, aspects of care, and indicators of quality. The weight times the initial score yields the effective (or final) score.

Resource E

Sample
Quality Assurance Plans

This Resource contains functional Quality Assurance Plans from two of the study sites, the MIT Medical Department (Exhibit 15) and Southeastern Health Services (Exhibit 16). Note that while the two "parent" organizations and their Quality Assurance programs have differing structures (one complex, the other relatively uncomplicated, as described in Chapter Three and Resource A), the plans themselves share many common characteristics.

Special items of interest include MIT's detailed description of reporting procedures, and SHS's specific attention to issues of confidentiality of information and potential conflict of interest.

Other programs use different formats. At the Washington Outpatient Surgery Center, the plan is a series of related but separate policies addressing specific Quality Assurance issues. At HealthNet, we have a relatively short written plan that references a user's guide of several hundred pages; the latter provides detailed instructions for all components of the AmbuQual Quality Assurance system. And at The University of Chicago Hospitals, there is both a detailed, lengthy organizationwide Quality Assurance plan and a more concise supplemental plan specifically addressing the assessment program for the ambulatory care clinics.

Exhibit 15. MIT Medical Department: Quality Assurance Plan.

PURPOSE:

The purpose of this plan is to establish a quality assurance program which will seek to improve the quality of care provided to all patients of the Medical Department. To achieve this goal, the program will:
1. Encompass all services rendered by the Medical Department.
2. Monitor and assess important aspects of patient care in an on-going, systematic fashion.
3. Identify and resolve problems which have an impact on patient care.

AUTHORITY OF QUALITY ASSURANCE PROGRAM:
1. Authority and responsibility for the quality assurance program are delineated in the Bylaws of the Medical Department.
   a. The Medical Management Board authorizes the Medical Director to establish and maintain a quality assurance program.
   b. The Medical Director delegates to the Quality Assurance Committee the authority to implement a quality assurance program.
   c. The organization, authority and responsibilities of the Quality Assurance Committee are defined in the Bylaws of the Medical Staff.
2. The Quality Assurance Plan defines the mechanism by which the quality assurance program is implemented.

ORGANIZATION OF QUALITY ASSURANCE COMMITTEE:
1. The Quality Assurance Committee is composed of representatives of the medical staff, the nursing staff, and administration. All members are appointed by the Medical Director for a one-year term.
2. The Chairman of the Quality Assurance Committee is appointed by the Medical Director for a one-year term.
3. The Chairman of the Quality Assurance Committee may ask other individuals to join the committee on an ad hoc basis when their areas of responsibility are discussed.
4. The Quality Assurance Coordinator serves as the committee assistant, and carries out all functions designated by the Chairman of the committee. The Coordinator is a voting member of the committee.
5. Committee meetings are held at least once a month.

AUTHORITY OF THE QUALITY ASSURANCE COMMITTEE:
1. The Quality Assurance Committee may request reports and minutes from all the services and committees regarding their quality assurance activities.
2. The Quality Assurance Committee may identify problems involving the quality of care provided by all services and committees.
3. The Quality Assurance Committee may make recommendations for problem resolution to all services and committees.
4. The Quality Assurance Committee may request documentation that appropriate action has been taken to resolve problems, and that problem resolution has been sustained.

RESPONSIBILITIES OF QUALITY ASSURANCE COMMITTEE:
1. Members of the Quality Assurance Committee provide assistance to each service and committee within the Medical Department in setting up programs to monitor and assess important aspects of patient care.
2. The Quality Assurance Committee periodically (at least once a year) reviews the programs established by each committee and service to assure that the following elements are present:

Exhibit 15. MIT Medical Department: Quality Assurance Plan, Cont'd.

---

    a. There is an on-going, systematic monitoring process, using indicators which represent important clinical aspects of patient care.

    b. There is a periodic assessment of the monitored data for the purpose of identifying problems in patient care.

    c. There is an effective mechanism to resolve problems within each service and committee.

    d. There is evidence that corrective action has been taken and follow-up plans have been instituted.

3. When needed, the Quality Assurance Committee provides consultative advice to assist each committee and service in resolving identified problems. This may include recommendations for further monitoring, improved interservice communication, and specific corrective action to resolve problems.

4. The Quality Assurance Committee monitors the problems to determine whether corrective action has been taken and whether there is sustained resolution. This is accomplished by reviewing the minutes and obtaining progress reports from each service and committee.

REPORTING:

1. Minutes are kept of all Quality Assurance Committee meetings. These are sent to the committee members, the Medical Director, the Executive Director, the Patient Care Assessment Coordinator, and the Medical Management Board.

2. The Chairman of the Quality Assurance Committee reports quality assurance activities monthly to the medical staff and to the administrative staff.

3. The Medical Director reports quality assurance activities to the Executive Committee of the Medical Staff and to the Medical Management Board.

4. The Chairman of the Quality Assurance Committee prepares an annual report summarizing the quality assurance activities during the preceding year. This report is submitted to the Medical Director and to the Medical Management Board.

5. The Chairman of the Quality Assurance Committee, the Quality Assurance Coordinator, and the Medical Director meet bimonthly to discuss the quality assurance activities of all the committees and services within the Medical Department.

6. A file of all data regarding quality assurance activities is maintained by the Quality Assurance Coordinator.

REAPPRAISAL OF QUALITY ASSURANCE PROGRAM:

The Quality Assurance Committee reappraises the quality assurance program annually to identify components of the program that need to be instituted, altered or deleted. Changes are made to ensure that the program is continuous, comprehensive, effective in improving patient care and clinical performance, and cost-effective.

Date of Issue: 12-11-80

Dates of Review/Revision: 1-14-82   1-13-83   1-05-84
                                     8-05-84   8-08-85   11-13-86
                                     2-18-88   3-09-89

Source: MIT Medical Department. Reprinted by permission.

Exhibit 16. Southeastern Health Services, Inc.: Quality Assurance Plan, 1989.

I. POLICY STATEMENT

Southeastern Health Services, Inc. (SHS), is committed to assuring a high quality of compassionate and comprehensive health care to its patients. It is the policy of SHS to employ only highly qualified and proficient medical and support personnel who are committed to a high standard of quality. It is also SHS policy to maintain its high standard of quality by the formation of this Quality Assurance (QA) Program.

II. PURPOSE

The purpose of the QA Plan is to structure a QA Program which continuously evaluates and monitors the medical care and services provided by SHS. The scope of the program will cover all aspects of medical care and the administration of services.

III. GOAL

The goal of the QA Program is to create a formal mechanism by which the quality and appropriateness of care can be evaluated and monitored on an ongoing basis. This mechanism will include methods for standards development, problem identification and tracking, and the provision for service improvements. The program will involve all SHS staff.

IV. OBJECTIVES

The QA Program's objectives are to:

1. Meet all local, state, and federal requirements to practice medicine in the State of Georgia.
2. Provide our patients access to quality health care services 24 hours a day, 7 days a week.
3. Credential all staff according to their profession and the requirements of their position at SHS.
4. Have all physicians and health care practitioners certified by their respective national boards.
5. Maintain safe, modern, and sanitary facilities, equipment and supplies appropriate to meet our patients' and staff's needs.
6. Assure confidentiality is maintained at all times and that a qualified Medical Record system is in place.
7. Provide all services in a professional, caring, and courteous manner by all staff.
8. Promote health education and preventative health care services.
9. Provide access to continuing education for all staff.
10. Practice peer review and monitoring of all services provided.
11. Monitor utilization of all services to assure appropriateness of care.
12. Investigate and evaluate all patient complaints.
13. Reduce the risk of malpractice and medical liability.
14. Provide continuous monitoring of all quality assurance, utilization review and risk management activities.
15. Protect the confidentiality of all QA, UM & RM activities.
16. Review the implementation and effectiveness of the QA Program annually.

V. AUTHORITY AND RESPONSIBILITY

   A. Governing Body

      The Board of Directors as the governing body has the ultimate authority and responsibility for the QA Program. The QA Committee is responsible for implementing the program and reporting its findings and recommendations to the Board of Directors.

      The program is administered by the Director of Quality Control under the Medical Director and the Quality Assurance Committee.

   B. Quality Assurance Committee

      The QA Committee is made up of ten members representing all departments of the professional staff and is chaired by the Medical Director. The Committee will meet monthly and have a scheduled agenda. Sufficient data will be made available to the Committee to identify problems and promote plans for improvement. QA indicators will be identified by the Committee to follow on an ongoing basis. The QA Committee will report to the Board of Directors quarterly.

      The QA Committee has the following subcommittees which will report their findings and recommendations to the QA Committee each month.

     1. Utilization Management Committee

        The UM Committee has six members and is chaired by the Assistant Medical Director. It will monitor the utilization of facility services, referral services, hospitalizations, and after-hours services.

     2. Risk Management Committee

        The RM Committee has five members and is chaired by a physician. The Committee will oversee morbidity and mortality, incident reporting, infection control, patient complaints, and safety.

     3. Medical Records

        The Medical Records Committee has eight members and is chaired by a physician. The Committee will identify and monitor the quality of our medical records system.

     4. Pharmacy and Therapeutics

        The Pharmacy and Therapeutics Committee has eight members and is chaired by a physician. The Committee sets the formulary and monitors prescriptive practices, pharmacy errors and medication reactions.

     5. Service Committee

        The Service Committee has ten members and is chaired by a physician. The Committee is responsible for the development, implementation and monitoring of the service philosophy and standards.

VI. COMMITTEE APPOINTMENTS

      Committee members are appointed by the Medical Director or his designee and approved by the Board of Directors. Members will serve a minimum of one year on their Committee and attend a minimum of 75% of all meetings. Members are eligible for reappointment each year. The 1989 Committee members are on page OC-4 of the Quality Assurance manual.

**Exhibit 16. Southeastern Health Services, Inc.:
Quality Assurance Plan, 1989, Cont'd.**

VII. CONFIDENTIALITY

All reports, findings, and meeting minutes are considered confidential information of SHS. Individual information which implicitly identifies health care practitioners or patients is privileged information and may not be disclosed outside of the QA Program. All information will be kept in the office of the Director of Quality Control in a secured file.

VIII. CONFLICT OF INTEREST

Committee members may not perform or participate in QA or UR activities of their own patients or other patients who may for some reason constitute a conflict of interest (e.g. family member or personal friend) which may affect their impartiality.

IX. IMPLEMENTATION

The QA Committee is responsible for the implementation of the QA Program with the support of the Department of Quality Control. The Committee will develop a 1989 work-plan for monitoring and evaluating patient services, identifying problems, and initiating solutions.

Individual departments will be charged with developing indicators of quality care and criteria to measure the indicators. Department staff will conduct ongoing monitoring and evaluation. Their findings will be reported to the QA Committee for further study if necessary.

The Board of Directors will review the activities of individual Committees to ensure appropriateness of the monitoring and evaluation activities and will follow-up to see that appropriate corrective action has been taken.

X. PROGRAM REVIEW

This program has been reviewed and accepted by the SHS Board of Directors at its January 1989 meeting. It will be reviewed again in January 1990.

Source: Southeastern Health Services, Inc. Reprinted by permission.

Resource F

Annotated Bibliography

American Board of Internal Medicine. "Clinical Competence in Internal Medicine." *Annals of Internal Medicine*, 1979, *90*, 402–411.

> Description of the major variables of clinical competence.

American Nurses Association and Sutherland Learning Associates, Inc. *Nursing Quality Assurance Management/Learning Systems: Workbook for Nursing Quality Assurance Committee Members*. Kansas City: Community Health Agencies, American Nurses Association, 1982.

> This publication is one of a series designed by and for nurses; this particular workbook is aimed at nurses in community health services. The manual provides explicit direction and examples regarding a five-step procedure for conducting Quality Assurance studies. The book contains worksheets, visual aids, and a reference section.

Anderson, J. G., and Benson, D. S. "AmbuQual: A Computer-Supported System for the Measurement and Evaluation of Quality in Ambulatory Care Settings." *Journal of Ambulatory Care Management*, Feb. 1989, *12* (1), 27–37.

> Describes the AmbuQual ambulatory Quality Assurance system based upon the ten ambulatory care parameters, which will provide a quantitative

estimate of the level of quality for each parameter and for the entire clinical care program. Developed by the Community Health Network Centers ("HealthNet") and Methodist Hospital of Indiana, in Indianapolis.

Batalden, P. B., and O'Connor, J. P. *Quality Assurance in Ambulatory Care*. Rockville, Md.: Aspen Systems, 1980.

Comprehensive overview of Quality Assurance systems.

Benson, D. S., Flanagan, E., Liffring Hill, K., and Townes, P. G., Jr. *Quality Assurance in Ambulatory Care*. Chicago: Joint Commission on Accreditation of Healthcare Organizations, 1987.

This book goes into considerable depth regarding the monitoring and evaluation process. Numerous examples are included. The examples come from all types of ambulatory health care settings.

Benson, D. S., Gartner, C. G., and Wilder, B. "The QIP Form: The One-Page Quality Assurance Tool." *Quality Review Bulletin*, March 1986, *12* (3), 87–89.

A description of an effective tool for tracking Quality Assurance problems. Computer adaptable.

Benson, D. S., and Miller, J. A. *Quality Assurance for Primary Care Centers*. Indianapolis: Methodist Hospital of Indiana, Inc., 1988.

Step-by-step pointers on how to use the ten ambulatory care parameters in a Quality Assurance program. Contains forty examples of indicators that can be used for monitoring Quality Assurance. Describes how to develop a Quality Assurance agenda based on the ambulatory care parameters.

Benson, D. S., and Miller, J. A. *AmbuQual: An Ambulatory Quality Assurance and Quality Management System.* Indianapolis: Methodist Hospital of Indiana, Inc., 1989.

A detailed, step-by-step description of how to use the AmbuQual quantitative Quality Assurance/ Quality Management system in the ambulatory setting. Includes the complete "generic indicators chart."

Benson, D. S., and Plaska, M. *Quality Assurance for Community and Migrant Health Centers.* Washington, D.C.: National Association of Community Health Centers, 1988.

Suggestions for implementing Quality Assurance in community and migrant health centers, based on the ambulatory care parameters. Specific chapters are devoted to a variety of disciplines.

Benson, D. S., and Van Osdol, W. R. *Quality Audit Systems for Primary Care Centers.* Indianapolis: Methodist Hospital of Indiana, Inc., 1987.

Written by physicians, this book contains eighty clinical treatment protocols, plus extensive discussion, examples, and sample forms for performing peer review and other clinical audit activities.

Benson, D. S., and others. "The Ambulatory Care Parameter: A Structured Approach to Quality Assurance in the Ambulatory Care Setting." *Quality Review Bulletin,* Feb. 1987, *13* (2), 51–55.

A description of each ambulatory care parameter and how it can be used in the ambulatory care setting.

Brook, R. H., Williams, K. N., and Avery, A. D. "Quality Assurance Today and Tomorrow: Forecast for the Future." *Annals of Internal Medicine*, 1976, *85*, 809–817.

Succinct review of definitions and discussion of problems related to quality assessment.

Coile, R. C., Jr. "Time of Transition." *Healthcare Executive*, Nov.-Dec. 1986, *1* (7), 15–16.

Succinct but fascinating look at the predicted future of health care in the twenty-first century.

Cunningham, R. "Trends in Health Care—Environmental Assessment." Paper presented at the Surveyors Conference of the Joint Commission on Accreditation of Healthcare Organizations, Chicago, December 1984.

Excellent consideration of the true nature of quality in medicine, and of the dynamic tension existing between health care costs and health care quality.

Donabedian, A. *Explorations in Quality Assessment and Monitoring.* Ann Arbor: University of Michigan, School of Public Health, 1980–1985.

A three-volume series on quality medical care and its evaluation. Very thorough and very basic. Donabedian is a recognized authority on quality medical care.

Flanagan, E. "Indicators of Quality in Ambulatory Care." *Quality Review Bulletin*, Nov. 1985, *11* (11), 136–137.

Suggestions of indicators that could be monitored.

Gonnella, J. S., and Louis, D. Z. "Evaluation of Ambulatory Care." *Journal of Ambulatory Care Management*, 1988, *11* (3), 68–83.

Article about a specific quality assessment technique, "disease staging," based on the outcome-oriented premise that poorer quality care results in a measurably less healthy sampling of patients. Begins with good discussion on quality measurement in general, including factors contributing to outcomes.

Guaspari, J. *I Know It When I See It: A Modern Fable About Quality*. New York: AMACOM (A Division of the American Management Association), 1985.

Fictional (and fun) account of a CEO grappling with the true meaning of quality and ways by which to assure it. Short, snappy, and effective.

Institute of Medicine. *Advancing the Quality of Health Care: Key Issues and Fundamental Principles*. Washington, D.C.: National Academy of Sciences, 1974.

Although older, this is still a fundamental and sound discussion of quality and Quality Assurance. The definition of quality in this reference is the one upon which we suggest all ambulatory care centers base their Quality Assurance programs.

Joint Commission on Accreditation of Healthcare Organizations. *The Joint Commission's "Agenda for Change."* Chicago: Joint Commission on Accreditation of Healthcare Organizations, 1986.

The document in which JCAHO specifically describes its "agenda for change" (highlighted in Dennis O'Leary's speech to the National Conference on Healthcare Leadership and Management, as noted below).

Joint Commission on Accreditation of Healthcare Organizations. *Sample Indicators for Evaluating Quality in Ambulatory Care.* Chicago: Joint Commission on Accreditation of Healthcare Organizations, 1987.

Suggestions for indicators that could be built into a Quality Assurance program.

Joint Commission on Accreditation of Healthcare Organizations. *Monitoring and Evaluation of the Quality and Appropriateness of Care.* Chicago: Joint Commission on Accreditation of Healthcare Organizations, 1988.

Detailed description of the Joint Commission's ten-step model for Quality Assurance program development.

Laessig, R. H., Ehrmeyer, S. S., and Hassemer, D. J. "Quality Control and Quality Assurance." *Clinical Laboratory Medicine,* June 1986, *6* (2), 317–327.

If patients are to receive the benefit of physician's office testing, reliable and high-quality laboratory results are essential. To achieve this, the physician's office laboratory must have an adequate Quality Assurance program. Several fundamental components of such a program are addressed in this article.

McClure, W. "How Good Medicine Can Drive Out Bad Medicine" (Tape). Speech presented at the 1987 National Conference on Healthcare Leadership and Management (sponsored by the

American College of Physician Executives and the American Academy of Medical Directors), Toronto, Canada, April 1987.

> Enjoyable and spirited speech outlining responses behind the development of McClure's "Buy Right" system for purchasing decisions in health care, in which quality is a driving force.

McClure, W. "The New Era of Medicine." Paper presented at the 1987 National Conference on Healthcare Leadership and Management (sponsored by the American College of Physician Executives and the American Academy of Medical Directors), Toronto, Canada, April 1987.

> Two background papers that together detail McClure's "Buy Right" health care purchasing strategy and its intended impact on quality in the health care system.

Maynard (III), E. P. *Statement of the American College of Physicians Before the Senate Committee on Labor and Human Resources.* 1984.

> An overview of Quality Assurance, with emphasis on peer review.

Meisenheimer, C. G. *Quality Assurance: A Complete Guide to Effective Programs.* Rockville, Md.: Aspen Systems, 1985.

> An overview of Quality Assurance methods. Of special interest to hospital and nursing personnel.

Nutting, P. A. *Methods of Quality Assessment for Primary Care: A Clinician's Guide.* Kansas City: National Rural Health Association, 1987.

> Contains several very good suggestions useful in any type of ambulatory Quality Assurance program.

O'Leary, D. "A Blueprint for Change" (Tape). Speech presented at the National Conference on Healthcare Leadership and Management (sponsored by the American College of Physician Executives and the American Academy of Medical Directors), Toronto, Canada, April 1987.

> Basically presents the highlights of the Joint Commission's "Agenda for Change," under which development of specific indicators will become a key in future accreditation decisions. The "agenda" also references movement toward outcome measurement, as well as the need for organizational assessment (in addition to purely clinical assessment).

Oswald, E. M., and Winer, I. K. "A Simple Approach to Quality Assurance in a Complex Ambulatory Care Setting." *Quality Review Bulletin*, Feb. 1987, *13* (2), 56–60.

> Article describing the genesis and operational mechanics of the system for ambulatory care Quality Assurance at The University of Chicago Hospitals. As stated in the title, it provides a relatively simple mechanism couched in a complex environment.

Palmer, R. H. *Ambulatory Health Care Evaluation: Principles and Practice.* Chicago: American Hospital Association, 1983.

> This is an excellent review of how to make Quality Assurance work. Many of the principles have been incorporated into this book. Good reading for centers interested in supplemental Quality Assurance material.

Payne, B. C. "The Medical Record as a Basis for Assessing Physician Competence." *Annals of Internal Medicine*, 1979, *91*, 623–629.

A review of criteria development and the use of the medical record for data retrieval.

Pirsig, R. M. *Zen and the Art of Motorcycle Maintenance: An Inquiry into Values*. New York: Morrow, 1974.

A thought-provoking discussion of what quality really is. The suggestion that caring is an important dimension of quality comes from this book.

Thompson, M., and Palmer, H. "Resource Requirements for Evaluating Ambulatory Health Care." *American Journal of Public Health*, 1984, *74*, 1244–1248.

The costs for data collection and analysis are considered from an academic perspective.

Van Osdol, W. R., and Johnston, P. E. *Quality Medical Records for Primary Care Centers*. Indianapolis: Methodist Hospital of Indiana, Inc., 1989.

Description of an effective primary care medical records system. Includes sample forms, policies, procedures, and a complete patient record. Several chapters discuss the role of the medical record in a Quality Assurance program.

Watkinson, S. A. "Economic Aspects of Quality Assurance." *Radiography*, May-June 1985, *51* (597), 133–140.

The subject for the Nicholas Research Award (1983), this paper shows that the operating costs of a basic Quality Assurance program are probably less than 1 percent of the overall operating costs of an average five-room X-ray department. Future professional implications associated with Quality Assurance are also discussed.

Watkinson, S., Moores, B. M., and Hill, S. J. "Reject Analysis: Its Role in Quality Assurance." *Radiography*, Sept.-Oct. 1984, *50* (593), 189–194.

A reject analysis for a twenty-six-week period in the radiology department of an oncological center. Highlights the variations in reject rates for different examinations as a function of time and discusses the role of reject analysis in Quality Assurance.

Williamson, J. W. "Health Accounting: An Outcome-Based System of Quality Assurance—Illustrative Application to Hypertension." In Nancy O. Graham, *Quality Assurance in Hospitals.* Rockville, Md.: Aspen Systems, 1982.

Explains the explicit role of a "health accountant" in a hospital and HMO setting. The health accountant, working with a clinical team that sets acceptable evaluation standards, measurement criteria, and intervention and education designs, participates in patient interviewing to determine the most appropriate educational and administrative measures.

References

Anderson, J. G., and others. "AmbuQual: A Computer-Supported Ambulatory Quality Assurance System (Scale Development)." Indianapolis: Original manuscript by a team from Methodist Hospital of Indiana, Inc., and Purdue University, 1988.

Benson, D. S. *Notebook of Quality Assurance Clippings.* Unpublished collection. 1989.

Benson, D. S., Flanagan, E., Liffring Hill, K., and Townes, P. G., Jr. *Quality Assurance in Ambulatory Care.* Chicago: Joint Commission on Accreditation of Healthcare Organizations, 1987.

Benson, D. S., and Miller, J. A. *AmbuQual: An Ambulatory Quality Assurance and Quality Management System.* Indianapolis: Methodist Hospital of Indiana, Inc., 1989.

Benson, D. S., and Van Osdol, W. R. *Quality Audit Systems for Primary Care Centers.* Indianapolis: Methodist Hospital of Indiana, Inc., 1987.

Bertram, D. "Physician Reimbursement and the Quantity and Quality of Health Care Services." *QRB: Quality Review Bulletin,* 1985, *11* (12), 364–365.

Boyle, J. F. "Address of the President." In *Proceedings of the House of Delegates — 134th Annual Meeting of the American Medical Association.* Chicago: American Medical Association, 1985.

Brook, R. H., and Hohr, K. N. "Efficacy, Effectiveness, Variations, and Quality: Boundary-Crossing Research." *Medical Care,* 1985, *23* (5), 710–722.

Cherskov, M. "Hospital Design Follows the Crowd to Ambulatory Care." *Hospitals,* Feb. 20, 1987, pp. 58–62.

Coile, R. C., Jr. "Time of Transition." *Healthcare Executive,* 1986, *1* (7), 15–16.

Crosby, P. B. *Quality Is Free: The Art of Making Quality Certain.* New York: McGraw-Hill, 1979.

Crosby, P. B. *Quality Without Tears: The Art of Hassle-Free Management.* New York: McGraw-Hill, 1984.

Cunningham, R. "Trends in Health Care—Environmental Assessment." Paper presented at JCAHO Surveyors Conference, Chicago, Dec. 11, 1984.

Donabedian, A. *Explorations in Quality Assessment and Monitoring.* Vol. III: *The Methods and Findings of Quality Assessment and Monitoring: An Illustrated Analysis.* Ann Arbor: University of Michigan, School of Public Health, 1985a.

Donabedian, A. "Quality Assurance: Corporate Responsibility in the 1990s." Keynote Address presented at the Multi-Hospital Systems Invitational Conference (sponsored by the Joint Commission on Accreditation of Healthcare Organizations), Chicago, October 1985b.

Donabedian, A. "A Primer of Quality Assurance and Monitoring in Medical Care." Paper presented at the Conference on Law Practice Quality Evaluation: An Appraisal of Peer Review and Other Measures to Enhance Professional Performance (sponsored by the American Law Institute and the American Bar Association, Committee on Continuing Professional Education), Williamsburg, Virginia, September 10–12, 1987.

Gelman, D. "The Megatrends Man." *Newsweek,* 1985, *106* (13), 58–61.

Guaspari, J. *I Know It When I See It: A Modern Fable About Quality.* New York: AMACOM (A Division of the American Management Association), 1985.

Honaker, C. R., and Robbins, M. F. "Quality: The Healthcare Watchword." *Group Practice Journal,* 1988, *37* (3), 10–14.

Howard, D., and Newald, J. "80% of Hospitals to Expand Ambulatory Services." *Hospitals,* Feb. 5, 1987, p. 74.

Institute of Medicine. *Advancing the Quality of Health Care: Key Issues and Fundamental Principles.* Washington, D.C.: National Academy of Sciences, 1974.

Johnson, D. M. "The High Price of Mediocrity." *Practice Life*, Aug. 1987, pp. 1 and 3.

Johnson, R. E., Freeborn, D. K., and Mullooly, J. P. "Physicians' Use of Laboratory, Radiology, and Drugs in a Prepaid Group Practice HMO." *HSR: Health Services Research*, 1985, *20* (5), 525–547.

Joint Commission on Accreditation of Healthcare Organizations. *The Joint Commission's "Agenda for Change."* Chicago: Joint Commission on Accreditation of Healthcare Organizations, 1986.

Joint Commission on Accreditation of Healthcare Organizations. *Monitoring and Evaluation of the Quality and Appropriateness of Care.* Chicago: Joint Commission on Accreditation of Healthcare Organizations, 1988.

Koska, M. T. "Push Is On for Ambulatory Quality Assurance." *Hospitals*, Sept. 20, 1988, p. 66.

McClure, W. "How Good Medicine Can Drive Out Bad Medicine" (Tape). Speech presented at the 1987 National Conference on Healthcare Leadership and Management (sponsored by the American College of Physician Executives and the American Academy of Medical Directors), Toronto, Canada, Apr. 1987.

McIllrath, S. "More Outcome Funding Sought." *American Medical News*, 1988, *31* (27), 1 and 44.

Morrow, R. "Outpatient Surgery." *Medicenter Management*, 1988, *5* (1), 19 and 22.

Munchow, O. B. "The Term 'Quality'" (Letter to the Editor). *QRB: Quality Review Bulletin*, 1986, *12* (9), 310.

O'Leary, D. S. "President's Column." *JCAH Perspectives*, 1987, *7* (7/8), 3–4.

O'Leary, D. S. "President's Column." *Joint Commission Perspectives*, 1988, *8* (1/2), 2.

Orwell, G. *Animal Farm.* San Diego: Harcourt Brace Jovanovich, 1946.

Palmer, R. H. *Ambulatory Health Care Evaluation: Principles and Practice.* Chicago: American Hospital Association, 1983.

Perry, W. E. *Hatching the EDP Quality Assurance Function.* Orlando, Fla.: Quality Assurance Institute, 1981.

Pirsig, R. M. *Zen and the Art of Motorcycle Maintenance: An Inquiry into Values.* New York: Morrow, 1974.

"Quality Assurance Activities of Administration." Memo to Quality Assurance Committee from Executive Director, MIT Medical Department, Jan. 14, 1988, p. 4.

Robert Wood Johnson Foundation. *Special Report (Number Two): Access to Health Care in the United States — Results of a 1986 Survey.* Princeton, N.J.: Robert Wood Johnson Foundation, 1987.

Robinson, M. L. "Sneak Preview: JCAHO's Quality Indicators." *Hospitals,* July 5, 1988, pp. 38–43.

Statland, B. E. "Caring for Quality." *Connections: Methodist Hospital of Indiana, Inc.,* Nov.-Dec. 1987 (Issue 25), p. 3.

Stein, J. (ed.). *The Random House College Dictionary (Revised Edition).* New York: Random House, 1975.

United Way of Indiana. *Hoosier Initiative 21: A Blueprint for Indiana's Future* (Pamphlet). Indianapolis: The Human Service Initiative, 1988.

Walton, R. "Workers Key to Methodist's Future." *Indianapolis Star,* Aug. 7, 1988, Section B, p. 1.

Ward, K. "Managed Care Experiences Growth." *Medicenter Management,* 1988, *5* (1), pp. 25 and 33.

Wildman, G. "Monitoring and Evaluation: The Joint Commission's 9-Step Model." *JQA: Journal of Quality Assurance,* 1988, *10* (1), 18–23.

Zak, S. J. "At the Cutting Edge: New Approaches to Quality Assessment (Part II — Ambulatory Review: The Minneapolis Demonstration)." In L. I. Solberg and others, *The Minnesota Project: An Innovative Approach to Ambulatory Care Quality Assurance.* Minneapolis: Minnesota Department of Health, 1987.

Index

A

AAAHC. *See* Accreditation Association for Ambulatory Health Care
Abnormal pap smears, 184
Academic programs, for Quality Assurance, 213
Acceptability, of care, 56, 60, 66. *See also* Patient satisfaction
Acceptance, of Quality Assurance, 211, 212; by physicians, 15–16, 107, 211–212
Accessibility, 56, 145, 223; to indigent, 59, 67
Accountability, 25, 53. *See also* Litigation protection
Accreditation, by AAAHC, 9; as aim of Quality Assurance, 25, 63, 65–67; by JCAHO, 7, 186, 225; in medical evaluation studies, 7; by NCQA, 9; as trend in Quality Assurance, 16, 22, 87, 141. *See also* Incentives; Sanctions
Accreditation Association for Ambulatory Health Care, 9
Acuity factors, 219
Administration, role in Quality Assurance, 25, 78–79, 80, 195, 196. *See also* Clout factor

Administrative/management review, 9, 97–98
Agenda for Change, 63, 98
Agendas and minutes, for documentation, 175, 181
Alexander, R., 37
Alternative providers, trend in, 10–14, 58, 114
Ambulatory care, trend in, 10–14
Ambulatory surgery center, as case study site, 36–43, 229
AmbuQual Quality Assurance program (HealthNet), 19, 48, 140–158; criteria and standards, 15, 120; data collection in, 67, 97, 126. *See also* Community Health Network, Inc.; Computerization
American Medical Association, 6
Anderson, J. G., 148
Anemia screening, 119
Annual review, of Quality Assurance programs, 186, 187
Appointment books, as data sources, 129
Appropriateness of care, 54, 91, 146, 197, 209; and cost, 58–59
Art of care, 11–12, 60
Aspects of care, 29–32, 96, 99, 100, 149

Assessment technology, 14, 17
Atlanta (Southeastern Health Services), as case study site, 36–37, 41
Attitude of excellence, 4, 65
Audits, as data collection devices, 131, 174
Authority and responsibility, of Quality Assurance program, 206–207
Autonomy, of provider, 212

B

Basic wellness, 12
Benefits of quality, 212
Benson, D. S., 93, 112, 120, 121, 148
Bertram, D., 91
Biller, B., 33, 37, 39, 64–65, 75, 83, 87, 104, 105, 111, 119, 122, 123, 133, 161, 163, 187, 222
Block sampling, as instrument of evaluation, 127, 138
Blood pressure, and outcome audits, 135
Boredom, and effectiveness of Quality Assurance, 104
Bottom-Up portion of Quality Assurance, 24–25
Boyle, J. F., 6
Breast examination documentation, 119
Brook, R. H., 117
Budget. *See* Cost; Financial incentives; Financial rewards; Resource allocation
Buy Right systems, 224

C

Cambridge (MIT Medical Department), as case study site, 36–37
Caring, and organizational competence, 61–62
Case information, as data collection, 127, 219
Case studies, 35–52, 229–252
Causally valid assessments, 142
Center for Policy Studies, 15

Centralized program notebook, for documentation, 181
Changing performance, by problem solving, 164
Chart(s), 6–7, 128, 129, 144; on computer, 216. *See also* AmbuQual Quality Assurance program
Cherskov, M., 10
Chicago (University of Chicago Hospitals), as case study site, 36–37, 43
Chronic conditions, effect of, on outcome evaluation, 92
Claims data, as data sources, 129
Clerical personnel, for data collection, 126
Client satisfaction. *See* Patient satisfaction
Clinical assessment. *See* Protocols and Standards
Clinical flexibility, and criteria and standards, 111
Clinical orientation, in Quality Assurance, 9, 71, 196, 215
Clinical performance measurements, 89, 107, 108, 131
Clout factor, 72, 80, 163; in Quality Improvement Plans, 156; as support for Quality Assurance programs, 17, 84, 141, 195
Cockerline, M., 34, 37, 66, 74, 107, 122, 162
Codman, E., 124, 166
Coile, R. C., Jr., 10, 63
Commissioning Quality Assurance programs, 25
Commissioning special studies, 81
Commitment of organization, to Quality Assurance programs, 17–18
Common aims, 39–40, 68
Common indicators and standards, 18–19
Common language, *See* Terminology
Commonality, 39–40
Communication technology, in Quality Assurance programs, 209, 214

Index